Advice (Upadesha) of a Modern Sadhaka:
Your Guide to the Path of Yoga, Kundalini Awakening, Self Healing, Self-Realization, & Life

Author: Darshan Baba

Moksha Gyan Books

Moksha Gyan Books

Darshan Baba email: omnamahshivaya8@gmail.com
Phone: +15756138137
siddha-international.weebly.com
siddha-life-mastery.com

Advice (Upadesha) of a Modern Sadhaka: Your Guide to the Path of Yoga, Kundalini Awakening, Self-Healing, Self-Realization, & Life

Cover Photo; Sunrise Over Siddheshwar, by Shambala Light Photography

"Just as there is a whole wonderful world to explore in the material realm of earth, there is also an incredible subtle world to explore and witness the marvels of!"
-Darshan Baba

Siddha Life Mastery

Online Courses

- Intro & Experience of Subtle Energy

- Ultimate Subtle Energy Mastery Course

- Ultimate Meditation Course: Siddha Jyoti & Nada Dhyana Kriya Initiation and Practice Instruction

Sign up FREE for an online course now at:
https://siddha-life-mastery.com

Introduction

This book is manifested as a result of the many emails and correspondence the author, Darshan Baba has received over the years.   There is One Humanity, and we are all like family.   Babaji's Grace is with you.   His prayers said "allow me to be the servant of the servants of your feet"... Service is real wealth here on Earth. Darshan always tries to be of service to anyone who reaches out through email and messages seeking advice, guidance, or simply support from another member of our Great Universal World Sangha Family.

This book then is a collection of questions, and the answers that Darshan provided to the seeker as advice, pointers to self-realization, sharing techniques for sadhana, and methods of self-healing.   Since many times we all may have similar questions it was decided to collect together some of these questions and answers as this book.   Also, it has been found that often some of the best information can be drawn out in Satsang through the seekers question in relation to the subject, difficulty, or apparent obstacles to realization they are experiencing.

In addition to the question and answers from

correspondence, this book includes some commentaries by the author at the time of writing, and some informative blog articles. Also, there is some new material from the author that seemed important to share with the readers of this book.

Spirituality, and "God"

Question: How do you know there is a God or Spiritual world?

Darshan's answer: "Spiritual" and "Material" are both concepts. Life is Undeniable. Consciousness is Undeniable. Energy - the Infinite Possibility to Experience Being, and medium of All that is *Seen* is undeniable. Without believing, or thinking, or imagining, but turning attention directly to *SEE*, from where is the Source of this Life. From where is the Source of this Consciousness. From where is it that All Perceptions and Experience (Energy) is *SEEN*...

Question: What is being spiritual?

Darshan's Answer: "Spiritual" is just a concept or idea

which implies a duality between "Spiritual" and "Material." They are one within the medium of Life. What people think of as "spirituality" is the remembering of the Essence and Intelligence of Life - Love (All Life as One). This Love (All Life as One) is Self-Knowledge, Intelligence, Realization. God is Love, each and every aspect, everything, all appearances of being(s) Integrated in One Perfect Wholeness of Supreme Being!

Darshan's Lineage

In Response to an email enquiring about Darshan Baba's Lineage, and the Siddha Subtle Energy Shaktipat Empowerment.

Darshan's Answer: Our lineage is Mahasiddha Gotra (Family of Maha Siddha's). Also, it is more about nurturing that same direct heart connection which is beyond the dry linear dogma of a line of teachers or identity with the outward forms or show of a spiritual "club". Darshan has always felt in the heart his Sadguru is Dakshinamurti Mahamunindra Maharaja - the King of Sages and Original first Teacher of all Yoga. It says in the songs of Mahamunindra Maharaj, by merely remembering

Him the highest or most subtle knowledge difficult to achieve is rendered easy, and Moksha is realized beyond a doubt...

In this way of being the student of a Sadguru in subtle form, Darshan has been guided to various living Siddha (Masters) and initiations under the direction of the Maha Avatar Munindra Maharaja, aka Babaji. Seeing in the unifying way of Babaji's vast influence, all these Siddha Masters are one family or all one lineage. We are all really one big Universal World Sangha.

Darshan does not fixate on a definition of our Lineage, as just like any of the games of mind it becomes a potential fixation of identity or ego. As you may have noticed in your travels in India and meetings with various Yogi's, many people think their way is the end all and be all. But Yoga is attained only in purity of mind and heart in which everything (including spiritual identities) has been burned or cleared to reveal the Truth which always is, which does not need to be created, or learned etc. But simply is the Ultimate Truth, while all other perceptions are relative and dependent upon That Infinity for a fleeting reflection.

The Siddha Subtle Energy Shaktipat Initiation is a reconnection directly to the Super Intelligent Light and Presence of All Perfected Masters (Siddha) combined.

The shaktipat is seen to be from the original primordial Sakti of Infinite Reality/Being. This Energy is Super Intelligent as the very Power of Everything *Seen*. All Energy, All Power as One Omniscient Energy. So, the Shaktpat channeled and transferred is not limited by "Darshan's" learning or attainment in Yoga, but is something specific to the receiver out of limitless possibilities of The Infinite Energy (Maha Sakti).

This body shares practices/sadhana for nurturing/integrating the Direct Connection and Guidance of the Shakti, based on each one's predilection. The ongoing sadhana is especially in order to further facilitate one's own direct connection to That Source of All. When we feel this direct connection to the Perfected Masters and Super Intelligent Energy of All, we can stop grasping or seeking externally. Or in other words, the sadhak can draw internally on the direct connection to the Guru principle (Tattva), the Perfected Masters, and Divine Energy (Divine Mother). Receiving guidance with the Infinite Possibilities, and Super Intelligence of the Limitless Being directly without needing to seek it from an external source.

What is Shaktipat?

Question: What is Shaktipat?

Darshan's Answer: Shaktipat is Yogic Initiation through means of Energy Transmission or gift. Sakti is Pure Energy or Power, unlimited potential. Sakti is a Super-Intelligent Force, the very medium of all the Infinite Possibilities of Manifestation or Experience. When Sakti is Transferred or Awakened through Shaktipat, the Super Intelligent Force of Sakti Herself (often personified as the Divine Mother) directs and guides the means and method of attaining the Supreme Form of Enlightenment.

Sakti as Kundalini (infinite potential with the image of a coiled spring ready to JUMP) arises through the Sushumna Nadi(Central Energy Channel) towards meeting Siva (Pure Consciousness Awareness), bringing all of our Infinite Power and Potential(Sakti) into the illumination of the Full Light of Consciousness (Siva) as Self/God-Realization...

Shaktipat Deeksha (initiation), and the post sadhana can indeed be a supreme means of attaining the Supreme Realization.   As it says throughout the scriptures and upadesha (instructions) of the Awakened Ones, that the Supreme Awareness can only be Realized by the grace of That Supreme Reality itself, and not by one's efforts, or cognition. The reason for this is that all phenomena are *seen* like reflections in the Infinite Medium of - Siva and Sakti's ever ecstatic marriage and dance. Pure Omnipresent Consciousness (Param Atman- Supreme Self - Siva) and Omnipotent Power (Sakti) to experience Being, and therefore anything else is just "a part" or an effect of That Primordial Energy Dance appearing in That Infinite Field. To Know the Infinity itself, the only means is by that Infinity, anything else is just a piece. In Shaktipat Traditions, your sadhana is to SURRENDER to Sakti to Allow Her to do all the efforts of sadhana for you. As the Super Intelligent Force of Shakti works to bring the Aspirant to Yoga, there is nothing that is overlooked. She- Shakti the Energy of all Manifestation knows exactly what Kriya's, Mantras, Asanas, Pranayama or other Practices will be of benefit to bringing you to the Experience of Yoga. These Kriya's and other practices take place automatically under the influence and guidance of Shakti Kundalini.

Actually, all sadhanas are simply clearing away obstructions of Kleshas (agreements about reality, ideas of the world) so that relative reality is out of the way to reveal the Truth - Ultimate Reality... All Sadhana is just preparing for SURRENDER. In Shaktipat Yoga Traditions, there is no maintaining of the delusion of self-effort (ego). Instead, there is the constant ideal of Surrender to the

Reality of the ever Illumined Being, leading to the Sure Realization of That!

Darshan's commentary for this book: Nearly every form of service offered by Darshan, the Moksha Gyan Books, Moksha Gyan Music, YouTube videos, Courses, etc. is considered a form of Shaktipat. All these formats have the intention of transmitting information as Energy (Shakti) beyond simple words or reading information. These various formats all offer Direct Super Intelligent Guidance through Energy on the Pathway of Harmony, Wholeness and Awakening.

Darshan spent years since the early age of Elementary school practicing methods of directly realizing the subtle aspects of Being. This is often called "internal cultivation". This has awakened various abilities or Awareness of Subtle Energy. After years of these practices, sadhana, mantras, meditation, and exercising Subtle Energy awareness and abilities, Darshan was further guided to integrate this through formal training with various Subtle Energy or Healing Arts. So, this transmission of Energy occurs automatically and naturally as a result of a Life relating with Subtle Energy.

When Darshan wrote/channeled the first book: *"A Self Attunement - Maha Moksha Healing"*, The intention was not just to write an intellectual reading. But, instead to create a reading which acted as an anchor like a portal to a Transmission of Energy for Direct Guidance, Healing, and Realization facilitated by the Super Intelligence of this Subtle Energy (Shakti). Since this first book every following book, and other formats such as the Moksha Gyan Music has been created with this same intention. Though the following books after the first contain more words, and information for practical application by the reader, the intention is still the same. The material acts as a focus for the conscious mind, while also receiving unlimited direct Guidance, and further direct connection with the Super Intelligent resources of the Universe for Awakening, following the pathway, and Harmony with the Wholeness of Being (Dharma).

Siddha Masters

Question: Who are the Siddhas or Siddhars?

Darshan's Answer: The Siddhas are Immortal Masters who achieved in ancient and modern times Perfection in all areas of Life. Not just "spirituality" or something "religious", the Siddhas are Extremely Advanced in many Technologies of Life including Science, Medicine, and Universal Society. Levels of attainment and mastery which the society of today (though mis-claiming to be more advanced) is yet to match...

Many of these Siddhas continue to maintain bodies for hundreds and even thousands of years not only through Yogic Mastery but also through Mastery of Medicine. Thus, as Powerful and Immensely Wise Beings with immeasurable experience in the ways of the World and Humanity, the Siddhars continue to interact with and Guide the development and course of events in this world.

The Siddha Sages from Ancient times have largely been hiding, in difficult to reach places, as well as in subtle forms, or in disguise such as pretending to be "normal" sadhus or beggars, average humans etc. Now the Awareness of Siddhas and the Possibilities of Being they demonstrate is growing and will continue to grow in the common knowledge of the world again.

We are going to be entering a Siddha Age - a "Golden Age" of Unfathomable Levels of Collective Harmony and Well Being through Greater Universal Wisdom (non-different from Loving Kindness).

Question: Why do you have pictures of (names of specific masters) on your webpage?

Darshan's Answer: There are pictures of Siddha's on the website because one is very fortunate to encounter the Darshan of a Siddhar. Pictures vibrate at the same frequency as the contents of the image in the photo. Thus, looking at the image of a Master is the same as having Darshan of the Master. Even just by looking at the image of a Saint, one begins to resonate with, become affected by their vibrations and can attain that same Level of Mastery through first Grace (Krpa), one pointed focus(Dhyan), Sraddha (faith), Bhakti(Devotion/Love), and Sankalpa Sakti (firm determination).

Darshan's Commentary for this book: We used to have a whole section of many different Masters pictures for download, printing, etc. Just for the purpose of people to have this Darshan of the Saints available and in their homes, etc. Now this section is no longer on the website. The question and answer was included in this book because it is an important tip. Gazing at the picture of a Siddha or Master you revere is a Very Powerful practice! It may be simple, but just because it is simple and easy does not take away from the potency of sitting and focusing on the Image of a Great Saint and highly Realized Being!

The first time in India, Darshan lived with Naga Sadhus for about a month sleeping next to Havan Kund of Kedarnath Temple. Near the end of this stay there with them, Darshan was sitting there gazing at a picture of Mahamunindra Maharaj. One of the Baba's who Darshan had lived with for that time saw him gazing at the photo and said, "this looking at Guru photo, same to same Guru Darshan". If you have studied any modern science experiments around metaphysics such as the many studies included in the book "the Secret Life of Plants", you are aware that this has been demonstrated many times. A picture is not just a picture, it carries the energetic resonance, and much more information than just meets the habitual seeing of the eye.

There really is no "mundane" world of dead or lifeless objects. Everything is pervaded by and appearing within the Field of Super Intelligent Energy. We really just need to become Fully Present, Clear of all these preconceived ideas and thoughts, then be Alert and Aware to *SEE*!

Who is Darshan Baba?

Question: Who are you? (Sent to Darshan's email through contact form on website)

Darshan's Answer: How do we answer the question

"who are you?" When SambaSadaShiv Alone exists - then "i" am an appearance of the never ending Maha Leela (Divine Play) and Infinite Possibilities of Maha Maya Sakti (The Great Divine Energy).   Thus Ultimately "i" am not, but in Reality there is only Siva (Consciousness) and Sakti (Infinite Power to Experience Being)...

Identity or Mis-identification?

Questioner: Identity is just another attachment?

Darshan's Answer: Identity can be an attachment... But really what makes up Identity is just an idea, stories, or bundles of thoughts.   Nothing we think of ourselves is really solid or tangible. In fact, it can change from one polar opposite to the next in a moment.   If you look into the subject matter, where do you find any real concrete identity?

Just contemplate it, look at your own identity, who are you...?   You may start to say you are your job, or your name, or you are the place where you live, or you are your likes...   But at any point have you really "identified" yourself?   Because all these things are things we do, or have, but they are not us. Even "your" name, it was picked out by your parents, before you had any concern for such things as names, so really, it's more theirs than yours...

So, who are you?

Guru Tattva (Essence/Principle of Awake Light)

Questioner: Aren't I my own best guru?

Darshan's Answer: That is not necessarily true at all. It could be very misleading. Because the ego is not the Self, and would make a terrible Guru who would never lead you to your Self.

The Guru is a Tattva, meaning a Principle like an archetype. The syllables mean the Light which Reveals, or When the Light of Awareness/Consciousness is Turned On, the "darkness" of ignorance naturally dissipates. When this is clearly understood, whether one has a "Guru" as a living teacher or not, one will understand why it has been said over and over in the ancient Upadesha(advice) of

Realized Masters that no one will ever attain to Knowledge, or Self-Realization without the principle of the Guru.

This idea, that "I", "me" is my own best guru has misled many into further confusion, and dissatisfaction... The Guru Principle is the Self-Realized, the Guru is a mirror. The ego can never fully realize the Self, in the same way that the Object of Perception is not the *Seer*. Everything, including every idea of identity is *Seen*, and is thus but a piece, a reflection, and due to its impermanence like an ungraspable mirage.

Only by the Grace of the Self itself is That One "Attained" or Known. This Light of Grace which brings the Awakening by means of what is already Awakened is the incomprehensible Tattva (Principle or Essence like an archetype) of the Guru. Only by Being can one know Being, everything else is but a projection like a mirage in a dream. The Absolute Nature and Totality of Being cannot be attained through any action, because it is the primary cause, the foundation of all *seeing*, how can it be caused by something which is *seen*.

The body is also not the Self. It is *seen*. We cannot even be truthfully said to be IN a body! The body is clearly *seen* WITHIN Consciousness itself, while Consciousness extends far beyond the body, and can even be experienced as Omnipresent.   Such as demonstrated in Remote Viewing or Lucid Dreaming.

Om Sivaaya Namah Om

What is the True Meaning of the Guru?

The True Meaning of the Guru is hard to reach even through meditation, as has been stated in the scriptures of Ancient India.   The Guru then is often misunderstood especially among westerners but also in India where "Gurus" are a common phenomenon.   This article should help reveal the True Meaning of the Guru...

The Guru you see, is a mirror, ideally a perfectly clear mirror.   It says in various scriptures that it is impossible to attain Knowledge or Perfection of Enlightenment in Self/God-Realization without the principle of the Guru. This is understood as True if you understand the Guru Principle.   The Guru is the Light of Awareness which removes the Darkness of Ignorance as is the meaning of the syllables.

In this way it certainly would not be possible for

illumination to occur without the Presence of the very Light of Illumination.   That is what the Guru is really, the very Light of Enlightenment (or even just all cognition) which reveals the Ultimate nature of Being.   The Guru then is not necessarily a person at all, and so Mastery or Perfection of Self/God Realization can occur without the presence of a "Guru" as a Person.   But not without the Very Light of Consciousness, which is the Supreme Self, and the medium of *seeing* or perceiving all the Infinite Possibilities of witnessed phenomena.

The Guru as a "person" is nobody at all, as they have surrendered completely to the Light of the Guru, which is the Supreme Self (Param Atma), and also Absolute Reality (Siva).   The Guru then manifests through that body or that "person" on a consistent basis as their entire identity has been surrendered to and thus merged in that Essence of the Guru Tattva.

The Guru is the Self-Realized...   The Guru then is a mirror, who can reflect back to "you" everything which appears to stand between "you" and realizing the Self. Surrendering to the Guru is surrendering to Self-Realization.   As the Guru principle embodies or represents the all-pervasive Omnipotent ONE Supreme Self.   That Guru principle (tattva) is the Light of Awareness which is the Life of All.   The ego is that which appears to divide or separate itself from the all-pervasive

Omnipotent indivisible Reality of the ONE.

   This is the simplicity of surrendering that ego to the ever-Illumined reality of the Self.   Pure primordial Consciousness is the source of all appearing phenomena of consciousness.   Avoidance of this surrender is why the principle of the Guru is cleverly misunderstood by the shape-shifting nature of the ahamkara - ego.

   "Your" consciousness is not a separate phenomenon of Consciousness from the all-pervasive original Omnipotent Consciousness.   Actually, there is not "your" mind and "my" mind, there is only mind.   This mind appearing in an all-pervasive Field of Consciousness with unlimited possibilities of experience including "yours" and "mine". Even "modern science" proves this if you have the Light of Awareness on to see the obvious in the data.   Without that Light of Awareness nothing can be seen at all, and it is not really clear to see what is in dim light.

   The Guru is the Light of Consciousness itself, which illuminates in perception all objects and experiences of cognition as they arise.   The Guru is Everywhere that Consciousnesses is then, which is even beyond and pervading all of space and Time.   Thus fully capable of serving each one in Self-Realization beyond a doubt.

Challenges

In Response to a Message about facing challenges.

Darshan Said: Namaste and pranams to the God/dess within your Heart!   Sorry to hear about the difficulty, but there is always some blessing on the other side!   This mind knows, because also recently went through a very challenging time in family life.   But during this so many blessings were received that were facilitated by the very ugly looking challenge, or that could not have happened without the circumstances.

In Response to an Email about facing challenges.

Darshan Said: Even what may appear as challenges is the Grace and conspiracy of the Universe for our highest good. That is why it can be important to practice stepping back from the immediate habitual and conditioned ways of thinking to see the world and Life from subtler and subtler dimensions of mind.   Then we witness the magic of life in more expansive freedom without feeling the need to wrestle with it and expect things to be a specific way.

After all, we entered this world naked with nothing, not even a name, and with the innocence of a child we spontaneously found joy and wonder Everywhere in the most simple things.

Mistreatment by a Co-worker

In response to a message about mistreatment by a co-worker, and ending with the questions: Can't our Angels help us? Why we are so helpless?

Darshan's Answer: Sorry for your difficulty Divine One! We are not completely helpless. You can try changing your own mind about the issue, and create a different programming about it. Then, sometimes there can be Miraculous change in the situation. If you completely change your own attitude, and self-talk about it, and there still is no change, realize that there is another message, or blessing to come from the challenge. And, realize also that what one says and how they act towards you had nothing to do with you though they may say it about you. It is projection of the "reality" in their own mind and heart. Someone who is lacking such love and kindness has their own issues to work out that are not yours to suffer, though they may project it at you...

Fear

In response to a message about facing some fear Darshan said: Prayers work.   Go back to your Self.   Back to your center.   Can that One be afraid?

The mind is a field of many influences. Everything is (appearing) there. "God's and demons are great givers of churning to the Mind..." -from old scriptures

Thoughts may whisper all sorts of reasons to fear. The thoughts are not you, and they can be liars.   You are the immovable field of Awareness in which all these appearances, thoughts, feelings, etc. arise.   You are a Beautiful Divine Being and you have nothing to gain or lose...   Life is living Life here...   Trust Divine Being/Life to Live you!   You are certainly so loved and supported by Infinity!   Watch amazing miraculous support continuing to manifest for you!

In response to a message in which while taking the Ultimate Subtle Energy Course many feelings from old memories that needed healing were starting to come out.

Darshan said: You need to continue to breathe as all this comes up to allow it to keep moving.   Don't let the arising feelings, memories, and worries overwhelm you as it comes back up to come out.   No matter what it is, it's just energy...   Just breathe...

Focus deeper and notice that whatever perception comes, you are still here.   Even if one is to face the worst of their fears, Awareness is still pure.

Stress & Anxiety

Question: How to prevent stress and anxiety?

Darshan's Answer: Breathe.   Center in awareness. Detach more and more from all that is *seen* "internally/externally" as the *Seer*, a pure witness.

If mind/emotions/heart etc. are too agitated or disturbed to do this, then repeat as much as possible a Mantra like Om Namah Shivaaya, silently or aloud, at all times and Everywhere.

Then as things calm and stabilize, look for the one who is doing this mantra, or who is doing anything.   Look for the one to whom agitation, stress, or anxiety arises. Look to *see* if the *Seer* of all phenomena arising in the mind, or apparently external can itself be seen... Can the *Seer* Itself be *Seen*?

Om, be at peace... May you recognize your own Essential Nature and as such be completely at peace!

Questioner Again: How to detach more?

Darshan's Answer: True detachment is not attained by trying to detach from something. That is only still focusing on the object of perception we wish to detach from. It is feeding the same energy in one way or another, keeping it alive. True detachment is attained by focusing on one's goal to such a point that the other perceptions fade out of focus, into the background, because our attention is so focused on the goal.

In such a case of focus elsewhere, we don't even necessarily notice we are detached. We are just focused on something else. Attention absorbed in something else.

It is the only way really to gain freedom from the extremes of the mind and emotional states. To be able to detach and dis-identify with them as a Pure witness. The One who is not coming and going with all the thoughts, ideas, stories, emotions, etc. Remain as the *Seer* of all that comes and goes...

That state of ultimate peace is your true nature, it does not come and go. Everything that is *seen* is in constant motion and change... but look for the *seer* itself.

"Can the *seer* of all this itself be *seen*?"-Mooji

Question: How to stay calm?

Darshan's Answer: Center in and stay with the breath. Breathe deeply, full connected breaths. Let the breath be calm and smooth and the mind/emotions will also settle. Detach from what is *seen* as agitation, disturbance, or emotions, and simply observe without trying to manipulate the feelings. You can also do japa (repetition of a mantra).

Attaining Peace of Mind

Question: How to have more peace of mind?

Darshan's Answer: Peace of mind is a most valuable attainment...

Simple practices are always good. Returning to presence through watching the breath again and again.

At any moment we can bring ourselves to a calm center of peace through staying with the breath. Practiced consistently over time we can exercise a greater habit of peaceful mind.

But, sometimes the only way for Darshan to establish peace of mind in the moment, is to just take a break, and transcend EVERYTHING! Any ideas of "identity", or thoughts/beliefs of the world, everything.

"Always not this, not this to both the formless and the formed. Only the Absolute exists transcending difference and nondifference." -Avadhuta Gita of Dattatreya, Swami Ashokananda Translation

"You do not belong to that which is composed of the 5 senses, such as sound and the like. Nor does that belong to you. You indeed are the Supreme Reality, then why do you suffer..." -Avadhuta Gita of Dattatreya, Swami Ashokananda Translation

Like this Darshan would Contemplate, moving beyond the senses, identity, and everything *seen*. There deeper and deeper within the subtle more expansive states of Being, Darshan has found there is always peace. Ultimately the only way to establish a lasting peace of mind here, is this greater in-depth experience and understanding of who we really are.

Naturally our identity and world come back, when we want. Sometimes even when we don't want, so we don't really need to be worried about losing everything.

We only have Infinite depths of greater Self-knowledge to gain... By taking a break to just let everything go and look beyond, even for just a moment.

Hope this spontaneous advice in the moment helps. Your message struck a chord with Darshan as well. As it just seems that so many are getting caught up in the drama, and collective noise in this time. So, we all have to remember from where we can really attain peace (within) and approach the world from this center of peace. No matter what the appearances may be in our circumstances.

Living in the "Modern" World or Society

Question: Why can't we just delete the monetary system? Why do we ruin our beautiful planet and why do we make people ill? Do we really have to accept the system we are born in? Living by this system goes against all my values, but Not following this system makes it impossible to live...

Darshan's Answer: This IS a loaded question!   One which Darshan can certainly resonate with.   In this time, the deception of this system likely goes far beyond what you are even currently aware of.

This is a time when the Knowledge, Wisdom, Teachings, and Practice of the Master's and Yogi's is critical.   It is the only way to have any decent quality of life here.   We need to realize the full potency of our Power, and the Nature of Being.

Then you can indeed live here without giving up your values, and can still have money flow in and through your hands, or choose not to.   Know the Truth...   Know who you really are, and none of the things of this world, no corruption can ever touch you!

One can also simply choose to leave behind this system completely and can still live.   In such a case it just takes the firm determination to break addiction to the grocery store, synthetic "medicine", the social system, media, etc. Food and Natural Plant Medicine Grows EVERYWHERE! One can learn how to identify these wild edible plants.

Darshan met the Master Maha Sambodhi Dharma Sangha Guru, who as a boy of 15-16 went deep into the jungle to sit for meditation 6 years without food, water, sleep, bathroom, etc. He has demonstrated what is possible here in this body, and time. Though such a pathway takes commitment, training of the body and mind, and practical internal as well as "physiological" preparation for such extremes such as forgoing food, water, and sleep.

Or as King Janak did, one can also choose to live in this world performing all the duties of life. King Janak lived performing all the duties of a King. While also never being "touched" by anything of this world as he was so absorbed in the Truth, The Infinite Being. King Janak is a perfect example from scriptures of India of a Jivan-Mukti, one who was liberated while still appearing in body to perform actions and responsibilities of a king.

Don't be tricked into giving up your values. Follow your heart and inner compass for Truth. Don't be deceived. Even if you should face difficulties, if you do commit to your Values, Truth, Kindness etc. You will attain a prosperity and happiness far beyond what anything material and temporary can bring.

Just don't worry about money too much. It comes, and it goes. Darshan's family has been living off of meager amount for months now [2016], while Darshan has had virtually no income. We lived homeless under a bridge for over a year, while this body worked full time hard farm work. Still we are happy, prosperous and ALIVE.

Hard times come; then always Good times will come again. The TRUTH of the Self is Infinite and unmoved by either. That Immortal Being does not follow the ups and downs of the world. There is always Peace in that expansive space and Knowing within!

Does this provide insight to help with your questions?

Feel free to email anytime you need anything!

Infinite Abundance be with you!

Self Judgement & Regret, Guilt, or Feelings of Making a Mistake on the Pathway of Sadhana or Dharma (Harmony)

In response to enquiry about the mind disturbing practice by doubts, feelings of self-judgement, or regrets for sexual lust.

Darshan said: God's only "Judgement" is unconditional

Love! Like the Great Saint Neeb Karori Baba is quoted to say, "Everywhere I look, I see only Raam (God), and that is why I'm always honoring everything...". You also are seen the same with the "eyes of God".

It is only through the misidentification with the personal mind which deludes itself with the thoughts "I am the doer" which seems to beat itself up with the never-ending chain of cause and effects called karma. But if you remain so focused on the Divine that even as parabda karma comes to fruit, it has no interest to you, or is seen secondary in the background, it would be like having no karma at all...

Even the greatest efforts of sadhana are not the doing of "me", they are by the Divine Grace Alone!

The little "me" that parades all over creation as BIG ME, poor me, alone me, misunderstood me, not getting what's deserved for me, better than anyone else me... Etc. etc. etc. is a powerful shapeshifter indeed! But actually, it is a very small part and role in actual reality which could never really be said to be the doer of anything... All of this is completely dependent upon the Supreme Lord of Consciousness and Infinite Divine Power to Experience Being!

Question: For some time, I was yogi. I was devotee of Babaji, but I did the wrong things and caused suffering to myself and others. I just ask if you can advise if there is anything I could do I am not presently aware of?

Darshan's Answer: Do not worry your mind! No matter what it is that you feel you have done wrong. There is nothing that you can possibly do which would end Babaji's Infinite Love for You!

Remember that Babaji has given His Promise of Moksha! Instead you will have to find a way to come to terms with, and FORGIVE yourself, to realize that you could not or would not make a mistake, except for out of ignorance. So, if you REALLY knew better you would not have caused such suffering. Therefor you can certainly forgive yourself!

What is called the "Judgement" of God is in reality UNCONDITIONAL LOVE! Recall the "equal vision" of Shiva! That demons and gods alike are seen with the same equal vision and Unconditional Love by Babaji!

Just go again for refuge (within). Take your heart and mind to His feet again, here now within. Give over all of yourself to His Love and Care. Allow the Light of Babaji's Grace and Knowing to penetrate into every corner and pocket of your being. Especially those places that you feel you need to hide, or feel dark, or closed... You know that He sees all anyways. So simply open up all these places baring yourself "naked" before this Light and Grace which is Babaji, and let Him in!

Taking Responsibility

Take responsibility! Manage your energy... IF you are giving the power away by placing blame on something else, then when you encounter difficulty you may find yourself fighting against or destroying those very energies that are helping your progress. For example, getting angry with your guides, angels, or helpers... Blaming them for your problems.

Perhaps going around your house ripping up pictures of the saints, angels, devatas, or guides - saying you don't believe in this stuff. Or destroying the manifestation list you wrote out and put up on the wall, saying "this isn't working..." But then you would be struggling against the very forces within your own being which are present for support and empowerment. When you lose faith in your tools just because of a challenge, then you are negating the opportunity for these tools to work for you in the moment.   Those are likely the moments when you most need your tools!

Do you want to feel better?   Able to accept and face the situation with peace and strategy?   Or are you (unconsciously) trying to work against yourself and create more difficulty, increasing the intensity of the feeling of struggle.

Challenges are part of life.   You would not enjoy it if everything were too pink, fluffy, and perfect for you. Think about it.

Would you watch a movie with no plot???   It would be dull and boring.   If you understand the nature of things, there cannot be a surprise when challenges appear in the cyclic world of change. What rises, falls...   Pleasure does not last forever, and so again pain will arise.   In the same way no ailment is forever, and good times will again arise.

The Self pervades this all holistically.   Every experience is a potential, and present within the Self. Each and every aspect contributes or integrates to one perfect whole.   All the pieces make up the totality which is the Super-Conscious knowledge of the Supreme Being.

There is no need to be overwhelmed by challenges and give up your power to face the moment.   Defeating yourself from the start with the wrong attitude.   You are a being of energy living in a world of energy. Infinite Resources of all knowledge, power, and abilities are at the tip of your breath in every moment! You can accomplish amazing feats! You can face any difficulty!

Worrying About Family

In response to a message describing worry and concern about family members, saying also they felt they were doing "penance" for "crimes" they had not committed.

Darshan's Response: Om.... Divine Brother, Service is the highest treasure in the world. To want to, and to offer selfless service to your loved ones is natural and beautiful. Just don't get mixed up in it. And, don't think too much. Allow the natural unfoldment of events to occur as they will whether we struggle with life or not.

Furthermore, you cannot change the mind of another. So, though you may feel that it is better for them to be near to you for proper care, if they do not agree and wish to remain as they are, then that is their own right, choice, and karma. Be at peace with their decision. Whichever results occur are theirs alone and not yours

Life is simply like this sometimes! It carries all colors, and flavors, light and dark, bitter and sweet... The Immortal Truth of Self remains unwavering and undisturbed among all of this constant movement of the relative perceptions. Life is never going to be all pretty and pink, and light simply because of Knowledge or Enlightenment.

The Truth is already the Truth, and all these appearances naturally arise and fall within That Infinity of Consciousness (Siva) with Limitless Power (Sakti) to experience Being. All of this is the Wealth of That One's Total Knowledge and All-Pervasive Omni Presence

Who is doing penance for something you did not do? Only the one who is not you... A false imagined Identity. This mind realizes that this kind of challenge is the most potent, with the caring feelings of your family involved. But the Truth remains ever the same, and Knowing this it is also fair to recognize that your family are also not limited to these forms. Their life-streams will carry them in whatever direction that is the best for them in their own Divine Pathway at this time. Even if this Divine Guidance in their lives is not ever apparent. This Divine Grace moves the Entire World.

Celibacy & Relationship

In reply to a message from a friend saying they had been practicing Celibacy.

Darshan said: That's strong of you to stay so centered in your commitment to your pathway and goal of celibacy even with still having opportunities as guys/gals are coming around.

You know that no one else will ever be able to make you happy, or truly satisfy and bring you lasting fulfilment. This fulfillment and happiness only come from within knowing the nature of Being. Staying centered in the Presence of Being, everything else can come or go and fall into place naturally.

It seems so silly to this mind that people focus their feelings of lacking something, dissatisfaction, unwholeness, or unhappiness on the idea and story that they would or could just be happy if only they find that perfect guy or gal.   The perfect guy or gal who's going to give them the satisfaction, wholeness, and happiness the mind is projecting out as needing to be sought in "the other".

The wholeness (fulfillment) of the Self can only be

found within. Here and now, with whatever is present. All the possibility of infinity is present. Otherwise it is lost in some phantom projections of the mind as "out there".

Follow the Heart on the way of Harmony (Dharma), and the Guru Tattva (Principle and Light of Awakening) Alone! Do not take for granted as real anything of this "modern" world, nor the many influences that can come in the mind which are like naughty spirits tricking us into giving our attention, belief, and misidentification to them.

The Light of All the Love you have ever sought in any time or place is shining within your own Heart! It's like this for all of us... we play silly games. We should always consider what it is that we really want. Being mindful if what we are seeking or working for in the moment is really in harmony or obstruction to our own Wholeness and fulfilled expression of Being...

Darshan's Commentary for this Book: Both celibacy and relationship are external appearances of activity (Karma) in Life. Freedom and Blissful fulfillment can come with Karma Yoga, or Union with Truth Beyond all appearances even while there is the appearance of action/activity. Whether we choose to be celibate or in relationship, we should realize that no one is ever going to be able to make us happy, whole, or fulfilled. If we can stop expecting this or projecting it on our partner then we will be able to have a more harmonious relationship.   If we are alone and can realize that this wholeness of Love is within, then we can attract a partner for relationship with the presence of Love, and healthy fulfillment of Self within. Or, we can also be content alone, realizing also that we are never alone, since we are All One.   Love = (All Life as One).

No matter whatever we may think one way or the other; doesn't it always seem that everything is following the Super Intelligence of Life itself? Why don't we just take refuge in That Supreme Being (Wholeness of Life) again and again, in every moment, every time we notice we have left That Infinity for another passing tall tale of the mind...

Relationship as Divine Worship - Powerful Sadhana

Often there appears to be a debate or duality between the Idea of a Monastic, or Householder Pathway regarding deep "spirituality", or intense devoted discipline.

Actually, there is no difference and the Same Teachings of Self-Realization apply no matter where one may be in life and what the apparent circumstances may be.

The Absolute Truth is not negated nor propagated by any relative truths. On the contrary all Relative Perceptions depend on the Absolute Reality of Self-Illumined Consciousness for their very Perception to occur. There is nothing which is outside of or excluded from Siva (Pure Consciousness and Sakti's (Power to Experience) Omni-present Dance. Even everything in relative perception bares the reflection of That Infinite Spinning Dance.

Relationship is a perfect example, and opportunity for Devotion, "self" (ego)-surrender, and Self-Realization in the Highest Ideal of Divine Love. This article discusses ways of bringing Awareness to the Opportunity of Sadhana and the Highest Self/God-Realization within Relationships...

"Love Everyone, Serve Everyone, Remember God"
-Maha Siddha Neeb Karori Baba

The simplicity of the Teachings of the Masters, the Unspeakable Knowledge of Self/God-Realization is related with perfect clarity in the quote above from the Great Master Neeb Karori Baba. Nothing has been left out, but to clarify Neeb Karori Baba says "Sab Ek" All One. This is the whole Truth, there is nothing that negates That.

Whatever you are looking at now is an opportunity to "Practice the Way". Sure, the Mind can shape-shift in Infinite possibilities of scenarios using anything as an excuse to avoid having to actually face Reality. Your partner, your family, and your children are an opportunity to, Serve, Worship, and Remember the Infinite ONE. Whoever it is, and even that inert rock thought of as unconscious - is an opportunity to cultivate and emanate an attitude, of Respect, Reverence, and Divine Unconditional Love.

The Truth of the All-Pervasive Supreme Self is present as the Light of Awareness within All. Anything you know about formal worship or reverence can be performed towards your spouse and children. In India there are festivals where Kumaris (young girls) and Vatukas (young boys) are dressed up and venerated as Gods and Goddesses in the way of formal puja and food offerings. The purpose of this Ancient rite is to remind us that Worship and Veneration does not belong only in Temples and Shrines. But that this True Divine Love for the One Seen in All, is the very means for transmuting and overcoming all our tensions and difficult circumstances in life.

The True Temple of the Supreme God is the Heart in You, in All. This is the Reflection of Siva (Consciousnesses) and Sakti (Possibilities of Perception/Cognition) which is the very Nature of Infinity. Self/God-Realization is certainly synonymous with Love(All Life as One).

Bring the Light of Awareness back to Itself; this is your job. Realizing the Truth and Love are your own Job, not for someone else to do, nor for someone else to meet your expectations or projections of. In every moment we find ourselves - that is the opportunity to practice Awareness, Choose Reality, the Simple Truth, and reflect That back as Love.

This is not limited to Romantic Relationship, but is every relationship to everything that is perceived as external (the other) to bring Awareness back to the Ultimate Truth and Reality of the ONE (Love). "SAB EK"-Neeb Karori Baba said! There is no "other" than God/dess, Siva (the Self) and Sakti (Power to Experience) in the Ever-Spinning Tantric Dance.

This is so Simple, so many words are not needed to elaborate! Every different branch of the True Teachings is the Same in Essence. The tricky or sticky part is that the Power of the Self to Experience Being (Sakti) really is Infinite and unlimited, thus we can keep spinning, dreaming, or projecting different scenarios of division forever. Seek the Awareness of and act in Harmony (Dharma) with the Whole of Life.

Darshan Baba in his travels, sadhana, and tapasya in India or in the west, would often meet people who would sadly say they felt that Darshan was lucky to be able to live a Life of sadhana. They felt they were not free to do sadhana as they had married and had families and felt it was too late. The mind can pick whatever it has at hand as the reason for dissatisfaction or dividing the Wholeness of Being. That is just a game in the mind. Darshan would always say that there is no difference, worship your wife and children as God/dess.

Philosophy is of very little use. Be pragmatic, taking up the practice of cultivating greater awareness to have the opportunity to choose rather than react. To remember the Truth and thus act with Reverence, Respect, Devotion, and Love to the Supreme Being. The only One with whom "you" are ever relating.

"Sab Ek, All One" -Neem Karoli Baba

With the Realization of this Supreme Truth how can there ever be any duality between "householder" or monastic practice? There is only the Simple Truth of Love, All Pervasive Awareness of Self.

As Haidakhan Babaji Said: *"Truth Simplicity, and Love"*

Shirdi Sai Nath: *"Have Patience, and Faith."*

Neem Karori Babaji: *"Serve Everyone, Love Everyone, Remember God..."*

Freedom

Question: What is freedom to you?

Darshan's answer: Discipline. Impeccability. Self (not ego) Knowledge. Ancient sages said that one's freedom was equivalent to one's discipline. The opposite of what many people think nowadays. Many people think: as long as "I" can get and do whatever I want, "I" will be or am free, but that is a kind of slavery to this thought ("ME", and "I want").

Remaining as the *Seer* rather than what is *seen*, detached as a Pure witness and mis-identify with the many objects of perception which come and go, thoughts, stories, feelings, etc. Remaining as the unchangeable, unmoving, constant Being rather than the ever-changing phenomena of all Perceptions.

How can any lasting freedom be conditional? When the conditions are not met or change the freedom will be lost... True Freedom is result of knowing what is the essential nature of the Self, and Life. That is what is important, use each moment to Realize the essence of Life!

Not anything we "know " is guaranteed against the wheel of Mahakal (Time)! At any time, this temporary form can be taken. Each and every moment we should use this opportunity to remember the immortal truth of Being

The possibilities of this Magic Field are endless... Take full responsibility for what you are reflecting in it, and never again dream a mundane world. Take a position of total surrender to that Infinite field of Maya as Mother of the Universe, realizing that She is the All, the only Reality, the only Doer or Enjoyer. Know All phenomena are Her dance of Maya, as such ungraspable, and Realize Immortal Wealth as True Freedom...

What is Karma Actually?

Question: What is Karma?

Darshan's Answer: Karma is something that is often very much misunderstood. This brief explanation should help bring clarity to the concept. Karma is often thought of as some out-there concept of "you did something good" so "God" or something is rewarding you, or "you did something bad" and now some Super Power is punishing you...   This is not really an accurate understanding of Karma.

Karma literally means action.   There are other words for action in Sanskrit, so Karma also is a particular aspect of action. Actions are never just an isolated incident. For example, there was the action of turning on the computer so now it is on and you can engage in the internet or all the other activities that go along with your computer. Earlier you got in your car and drove home from work so now you are Home.   That is Karma - it is very Simple.

Sometimes the effects of our actions may not always be apparent, as there are infinite dimensions to Being. Some of these aspects of Being are very subtle, or perhaps have been out of the scope of normal habits of perception. For example, there is the data of the numerous experiments that have been done which show that by having a certain group of people meditating, the whole community or town became more peaceful and crime rates dropped. Even those that are not meditating are affected by the actions (Karma) of the group. Actually, the group is affected by the experience and Awareness (such as meditation) of each ONE! This is also Karma working in the same way as the clearly logically seen way of "I put the pizza in the oven and so now it is hot" or "I am always loving, kind, and of service to everyone, so naturally everyone is the same towards me when I am in need"...

In Carlos Castaneda's Don Juan Books - Don Juan Said: *"Either work to make yourself (the world) Happy or miserable, the work is the Same..."*

The Yogi's Understanding of Renunciation

Renunciation is the Essence and the Simplicity of the Supreme Teaching. However, Renunciation is very easily misunderstood, especially in India and other places where an outer lifestyle or show of renunciation is a common part of the culture.   This article should clarify what the Yogi's Really meant by and Knew as the experience of Renunciation...

The Great world famous "Hugging Saint" Amma has a quote from the "Upanishads" in the front or back of many if not all the Books in Her Name.   This quote is frequently translated as "Through Renunciation alone, Immortality is achieved..."   What does this mean? *

The implication of Renunciation and full Understanding is Synonymous with Freedom (Moksha) and Self-Realization.   This True Renunciation has nothing to do with wearing robes or living a Monastic Lifestyle at all, nor is this Renunciation negated by such a lifestyle - as it cannot be negated by what is referred to as a "Householder" Lifestyle.   The Simplicity of True Renunciation - is an inner experience in which one can let go of what is perceived to be true about Reality to simply let Ultimate Truth and Reality to Be as it is.

Consider this with logic and Reason.   If you can just let go in any given situation (and still act) without trying to control, project, or wrestle with the outcome of the given situation - well then you are just free right?   If it needs to be like this, or this one is good and that one's not right - well then if those conditions are not met things did not work out?

We came naked into this world. Spontaneously Consciousness arises with so many Possibilities of Experience, but actually there is nothing here that you can really call your own. Every little bit of it is a Gift of the Wonders in the Infinite Experience of the Self (Pure Consciousness). Renunciation is just the simplicity of this Understanding; I Am Infinity, everything else is arising within That Totality of One Supreme Self (Param Atman / Siva) with Infinite Power (Sakti) to Experience the Self.

What can take away from That Infinite Wholeness then? Then if one is always established in this Ultimate Truth of Self, they can act in this world or not, practice austerities or not; but what could possibly add or take away from the Ultimate Immortal and Immutable Being who is the Very Infinity in which all Worlds and Possibilities arise?

"Through Renunciation alone immortality is achieved..."
-Kaivalya Upanishad

There are many stories in the Scriptures and Teachings of Ancient India that tell of beings practicing Great Tapasya (austerities) such as meditating on the Powerful Maya Bija Mantra for hundreds or thousands of years. After being pleased with such Extreme Practice the Deity of veneration appears to grant the aspirant a boon.

"I want to be Immortal" Says the completer of Extremes in self effort to attain their goal. The God/dess then proclaims a common statement which "protects" the Truth from those who are incapable of Surrendering the ego to Reality. "Anything that is born must die, that is a fundamental truth of creation..."

The Ultimate Truth of the One Supreme Self is Immortal, Omnipresent, and Omnipotent Being. There is nothing separate from That One Infinity, the Power of the Absolute is indeed Ultimate. Surrendering all relative reality to That Ultimate Truth is Renunciation. It says in the Yogic Teachings who Realizes this State Becomes One with God, or Goddess, the Creator and Destroyer of the Entire Universe.

The Great Ego lusting for this Great power and deluded with the meaning of these Teachings practices Yogic Techniques with great zeal but can never become That Infinity for it (ego) is only a piece. Surrender, Renounce, Yagya (Sacrifice) just let go and be Free. The Power of the Self can certainly continue to Shine. The Infinite Possibilities of Supreme Undivided and All-Comprehending Consciousnesses can certainly be your guide in all aspects of Life.

Dattatreya the Great Siddha Sage, and embodiment of Renunciation said:

"Renounce the World in every way, Renounce Renunciation in every way. Renounce the poisons of renunciation and non-renunciation; the Self is pure, Natural, and Immutable." -Avadhuta Gita of Dattatreya, Translation Swami Ashokananda

As long as we are thinking about reality, this is an experience from a limited dimension of knowing. If we can just let go of whatever we may believe, think or expect reality and our "selves" to be then perhaps we can have Clarity of Awareness to See, otherwise we can only see through the contents of mind. This should make it clear why what is meant by the Yogi's as Renunciation is indeed a preliminary to Self-Realization, for how can we know the reality of the self if we habitually invest in thinking and believing the self is something else?

Established (Always Identified) with the Immortal, Unchanging, and Ever Perfect Truth of the Supreme Self, it should be clear that it would matter very little if one is living in a House or Under a Tree. Everything is Perfectly Liberated and Taken care of as it stands within the Supreme Being, which is actually the Only Unchanging Reality which cannot be negated - the Super Conscious Mind (Turiya).

In the Conscious and Subconscious Mind, the relative truths there are constantly changing, never of consistent values. One's own idea of self and the world can be completely different and inconsistent even from moment to moment in the experience of the Sub Conscious and Conscious Mind. The Super Conscious Mind Remains the Same Regardless as the various experiences arise and fall because It is the Very Infinite Medium of Consciousness in which all the Infinite Possibilities occur.

Renunciation then is Synonymous with the Supreme Teaching of the Simple Surrender of all relative reality to the Realization of the Absolute Reality. It is not implying a dualistic concept of life "in the world" or "outside of worldly life"(monastic). The True Realization of Renunciation is a Unification of the Experience of Consciousness through relaxing and releasing the need to divide and "pit" aspects of mind against each other; this as opposed to that.

True Understanding of Renunciation is Ultimate Freedom, Liberation, known as Moksha. It's as Simple as just letting go to let Consciousness Be.

*These short statements from the Illumined Experiential understanding of our Enlightened Preceptors have many levels of meaning and Wisdom which the aspirant of Self-Knowledge gains through deep introspective (beyond rational thought) and experiential relationship to the teaching. Even if these things are "thought" to be understood rationally at first glance, there are Infinite Levels of Wisdom to the Sages Realizations, and these short statements are packed with several Dimensions (or levels) of meaning.

Discovering Your "Higher Purpose" in Life

Question: What is my higher purpose?

Darshan's Answer: To discover your "higher" purpose, you will want to deeply connect to your inner being, your "central axis of being", called the central channel, or sushumna...

Here is a simple practice you can do.   Settle into the breath.   Then center yourself deep within.   Imagine or feel that there is a line of energy within you along, the spinal column.   Imagine or feel that this line goes all the way into the infinity below you, and above your head.

Now, imagine that this line naturally pulls itself gently taught from the infinite ends above and below, aligning this channel of your incarnation line within the body. Sense into this deep aspect of being.

Simply by doing this, your life will naturally start to align with your life's purpose, and CHANGES may occur. You may or may not feel directly during this exercise a knowing of your purpose, or simply a greater feeling and sense of purpose.   Regardless of this, when this channel is in alignment, your life's purpose will naturally manifest in life, and will become more clear.

How Long will the Pathway of Sadhana Take?

Question: I have been on the meditative paths since 1988 (Buddhist samatha, insight, sound current, Sant mat, and finally mudrashram).   I was initiated into kundalini shaktipat last Feb. 2017 and the kriyas now happen incessantly... ...Since I have limited time to add other meditations, I would like to know how long your systems might take to awaken these inner senses.   Also, which

senses would they awaken (inner seeing, hearing, ...
astral travel, kundalini...)?

Darshan's Answer: The timing is always dependent on
the student's Intensity of Practice, accumulated results of
past actions (karma)/attachment to this karma/action
dimension of experience, and kleshas (knots in energy
field and stuck impressions of "identity" world etc.).

You already have a great combination of practices,
don't give up.   Only burn with greater Intensity and you
will reach the "Goal" faster.   The Ultimate Truth and
Reality is Illumined Pure Awareness, "you" are only a
mirage.

That is a key to cutting through everything quickly.
Focus on That.   In this way Shamatha (Calm
Abiding/Mindfulness) meditation is going to be your
Powerful Key in combination with your other practices....
Because as you noticed it's like jumping over the mind and
its many games to place Energy and Focus directly in Pure
Awareness.

Use this all the time, while you are practicing with
efforts such as bija mantra as well.   In the background go
direct into calm abiding in awareness.   So, for example,
when you are in bija mantra practice, look for who is
doing the practice, where is it coming from? where is it

going?   Notice that all the many movements of perception no matter how strong or what they are, they are of the same nature, and medium of perceptions, while Pure Awareness always remains the Same.

Everything else is coming and going.   But Awareness Always Remains!

Everything will get clearer and clearer through the other practices like Kundalini Kriyas (spontaneous) Super Intelligent Divine Mother Sakti's Guidance, Bija mantra, etc.   These will consistently burn away and clarify the field of mind which is being like a filter through which life is being experienced.   This will make it easier and more Natural to abide in the Pure Awareness called the Self in Yoga pathway.

Don't be attached so much to little attainments or abilities, it's just a projection of mind.

Instead focus more and more on the Ultimate Reality of Being...   No matter what you are doing, loosen the hold of delusion that "you" are doing anything at all.

You can do mantra internally with every breath, or throughout the day.   Increasing the speed with which you can reach your Goal(s).

The system this body relays through this course

(Ultimate Subtle Energy Course) is a simple way of stilling the mind to notice Subtle Energy and Focus on that All-Pervasive Sakti which is Super Intelligence itself to allow this Energy to guide each student directly however is needed. If you are already having spontaneous Kundalini Kriyas, the effects of Sakti are not even so subtle anymore. Just surrender to this Divine Force, Trust and Have Faith, focus on the Feeling, and whatever Perception of this Energy you have. Allow "Her" (Shakti) to Guide you as a Super Intelligent Divine Mother.

Don't allow your mind to trick you, every thought is just a thought. Even "I haven't awakened subtle inner senses yet." or "I'm not progressing fast enough," or "I still feel Lust". You don't necessarily have to believe any of these thoughts... Turn within and look directly to *see*: Who believes them?

May this Inspire and Guide!

Sadhana Practice

Question: Is the limit of sadhana to two times per day any precaution?

Darshan's Answer: Sadhana is often recommended to be practiced in the morning and the evening in order to fit around the busy schedule of most people in the employed world. You can perform as much of meditation practice as you like, especially since you have been practicing consistently for a while now. You can also increase pranayama practice, but it is the kundalini pranayama which should be gradually increased in order to build up energetic capacity in a sustainable way.

When the mind really settles into this stillness and equilibrium, that is the time to really "dive in" or fold mind in on itself, simply look for the meditator, or look for what is mind, what sees mind, and "can that seer be seen"... In other words, now that the fluctuations or objects of consciousness have calmed and settled notice the Infinity of Consciousness (Siva).

Question: Tried to send a telepathic message to you and felt something coming back, but I was not sure if it was genuine contact. (Also describing some subtle experiences from practice of sadhana, in relation to seeing the perceived identity).

Darshan's Answer: Sure, the message you received is good, the more mind a can detach from expectations, projections, and its contents, the clearer one can be to receive any sort of message or guidance from any being, and directly from infinity...

Notice how when you see "your perceived identity", the minds contents etc. how they are not exactly graspable or tangible either, as the meanings, values, or appearances are constantly in motion or changing into something else. The view of who you think you are can change to a completely opposite view in an instant from the right storm in mind, etc.

"Can the seer of all this be seen..." Is a contemplative question, what "Mooji" calls one of his piranha questions, because it eats up everything else, instead of focusing on the many concepts and contents of perception, we look for the root of all perception... When you notice the feeling of something subtle and still which is seeing everything and turn to look but see nothing, that is the meaning of "emptiness"... This kind of thing cannot be adequately shared through words as you can see the experience transcends words, one must discover this through direct encounter...

Siddha Jyoti & Nada Dhyana Kriya

Question: General Inquiry about Siddha Jyoti & Nada Dhyana Kriya (concentration technique utilizing Subtle Light and Sound as subtle object of focus)

Darshan's Answer: Sadhana with focus on the Subtle Energies such as Nada Sound and Subtle Light of Maha Shakti in these subtle forms can be useful as a pragmatic exercise into/and use of these subtle dimensions of our Being... it is like working in through layers of perception like the layers of an onion

So, in this way you work "inward" to broader dimensions of Being... For example, in "watching", Feeling, and merging with the Prana Shakti - there can arise an experience of Oneness with all Life since this Life Energy or Prana Shakti is One in All.

You may have already been noticing, or having experiences of this Ocean of Subtle "Sound" and/or "Light" (it "looks", "sounds", "feels" the same, as it really transcends the limits of the outward senses) arising in your meditation/sadhana and sadhana of daily life. It is not easy to describe these subtle dimensions of experience through the limits of spoken language.

It is best to receive this Siddha Jyoti & Nada Dhyana Kriya as a direct initiation. In order to guide the focus and experience of these Subtle "Realms", and to transmit through Subtle Energy a package of Information/Transmission/Download. As Darshan has also received from "Seers" along his path. Contained within this transmission of information as Energy is what would "equate to 200 years of meditation"- (as one of the Yogi's Darshan Baba received a Transmission/Initiation like this from had said). The Super Intelligent force of this Energy (Shakti) then guides and unravels itself in time through means of focus on these dimensions of Subtle Light and Sound Energy.

Question: I have a question regarding the Jyoti (subtle light) and Nada (subtle sound) sadhana. Is it to be done after the other sadhanas or separate or does it not matter at all? Most of the time I don't see lights nor hear sounds.

Darshan's Answer: The Siddha Jyoti & Nada Dhyana Kriya, can be practiced all by itself or in combination with Contemplation (Enquiry). When practicing the concentration, remember to stay as a pure witness (the seer). Don't try to manipulate the subtle light or sound, imagine it, figure out what it means or what you can do with it etc. Just observe the Subtle Light and Sound show.   The Super Intelligence of the Light and Nada Sound itself will guide what is seen within the field of perception.   Remain as the Seer, a pure witness of whatever arises.

This is the exercise of detachment from what is seen, to be more and more centered in the Unmovable state of the Seer which is not affected in any way by what is seen.   If you feel an identity with something which seems affected by what is seen, then you can notice that is also appearing in the realm of perception.   It is also seen.   Noticing this, sink deeper into Being, stay as a witness.

When combining the concentration practice (Siddha Jyoti & Nada Dhyana Kriya) with contemplation, simply look for the very roots of the Perception of Subtle Light and Sound.   Once can contemplate, where is the Subtle Light or Sound coming from?   Or, who is seeing this Subtle Light and Sound? Remember this contemplation is not a thinking about the subject.   The contemplation is a direct looking with Awareness.   Like following along one end of rope which has been found, looking for the source, you are not thinking about it, you are directly looking with Awareness.   This is again the use of the Seeing Power.

If you have difficulty concentrating on the Subtle Light (Jyoti) and Subtle Sound (Nada) or don't perceive these you can simply concentrate on the Jyoti (Light) Mantras given to you during the Siddha Jyoti & Nada Dhyana Kriya Initiation, or the online course at siddha-life-mastery.com. You can also concentrate on a mantra like Om Namah Shivaaya. If you are repeating mentally a mantra, remember to really focus awareness on the mantra to exercise this ability to concentrate. You will notice in time that the repeating of these mantras will increase your Awareness of the Subtle and will seem to call or draw out the perception of Subtle Lights and Sound.

Contemplation

The nature of contemplation is a direct inquiry with Awareness and the *Seeing* Power. Not thinking about a subject, but instead looking directly with Awareness to *SEE*. Such as from where do the thoughts come. Or where does the body manifest from. Padmasambhava's pointing "without concentrating on the object of meditation, look for the meditator."   Mooji's "Can the Seer of all this itself be Seen?".   Dattatreya "you do not belong to that which is composed of the 5 objects of sense such as sound, nor does that belong to you. You indeed are the Supreme Reality, why then do you suffer." In this way it becomes a direct entry to Pratyahara and even Samadhi/Absorption...

The *Seeing* Power

In stillness we can reach the potency and power of the moment. In this full presence we can catch the vibrancy of Energy dancing in the stillness. In the infinite space of the moment, there the Super Intelligent Energy of the Universe spirals in ecstasy. A shining and shimmering world of light!

Darshan cannot emphasize enough, the importance of discovering and utilizing the *Seeing* power! The ancient keepers of Knowledge of India were called Rishis - *Seers*. The ancient medicine people, intermediaries between the "gross", "subtle", and multiple dimensions of Life were *Seers*. The men and woman of Knowledge of ancient Mexico as portrayed by the Carlos Castaneda "Don Juan Books", and other "Toltec" books such as by Don Miguel Ruiz, were also called *Seers.*

Everything perceived, all witnessed phenomena are *seen*, not in the "physical" visual sense. But by the light of Awareness, or the Illumination of Consciousness. Go into your *Seeing* power. Un-moved by all that is *seen*, settle deeper and deeper into this *Seeing* power, and *See* more and more. Aware of the bigger picture in direct silent knowing of this pure witnessing or *seeing*. All phenomena arise within the Infinite field of Awareness and Consciousness. Thus, *Seeing* can be omniscient and omnipresent, illumined in direct knowing of the Super Intelligence of All-Pervasive Awareness.

1. Remember always to become centered, present, and Aware in the moment through the Breath.

2. Learn to stay AS Awareness centered in the *Seeing* Power itself.

3.Then you can remain detached from All that is Seen as the Seer Itself...

We can notice if we can become Present, Alert, and Aware that *EVERYTHING* is *Seen*. Everything that is *Seen* is in a constant state of motion, whereas the *Seer* always remains motionless...

If I think I am this or that, whatever it is it is *Seen*. Who *Sees*? Am I the one who is *seen* coming and going, if so, who remains to see the thought or feelings come and go, or change? Stay as the *Seer* Itself. Thus, one can *SEE* more and more even merging with Pure Omniscient and Omnipresent Awareness while being completely

Unmovable by what is *Seen*... This is the Divine Play of Consciousness, with Infinite Power to Experience Being!"

Seeing Subtle Energy

Question: Have been working with the techniques in the Ultimate Subtle Energy Course, and, maybe can see something, but not sure.   Any suggestions?   I *feel* a lot of things, but I would like to see them too.

Darshan's reply: The point of these exercises is just to allow the eyes to relax, and still, while bringing awareness to these subtle "visual" phenomena which can still be *seen* in motion while the eyes are undistracted with the habit of focusing on a gross "material" world. The thing is that this "*seeing*" transcends what we think of normally as the sense of vision, or any of the senses.   So, when you more clearly "*see*" the energy which you "*feel*" you *see* it the same why you *feel* it.   As subtle sound it "sounds" the same way that it "looks" and "feels".   The senses seem to blend and are transcended in a way that information is not limited through a divisive filter.

The dark room exercise (gazing in a dark room) can be

65

the easiest. As we really just want to remove the distraction of our normal habit to keep looking at the density of our gross material world. Then we just remain aware and witness. Commonly we have gotten in the habit of "writing out" subtle perceptions because we learned that they were unimportant or not real. So even in a completely dark room where you can't see anything physically, the mind will often skip over the subtle perception by this habit. The remedy is stillness, and increased awareness through the breath. The number one way we habitually skip over super perception is through divisive/limiting thinking or perception and constant motion/staying busy.

So even if we sit down cross legged with eyes closed, the mind will tend to go here and there and everywhere. And, for most people who have not made this stillness a habit, the mind will already have them up and moving and busy engaged in some other activity.

In this same way you don't really want to try too hard in *seeing* the energy, but instead practice the exercises as an experiment. Simply allow, and *notice* what you witness without looking too hard for it, or thinking that you can or can't see energy etc.

Breathe, still yourself, and just allow your awareness to witness. Focus in on how you CAN *feel* the energy, rather than where or how you can't...   As you focus in on the awareness of the subtle, the subtle perception grows. For example, if I simply focus on the subtle light that I "*see*", then without trying the subtle sound that I "*hear*" comes more into focus, grows louder, and more tangible.

Likewise focus on the *feeling* of Subtle Energy Information however it shows up for you...   This information will reveal itself more and more to you in a myriad of ways just by paying attention.   And, by making it a habit of perception viewed as important again.

So, the main tip for you is to focus on how and what you can *feel* or *sense* while practicing these techniques. As you bring focus to the subtle it will become less subtle and easier to perceive in other ways.   Also, you can start with focus on what you can *feel*, then ASK this Energy as a Super Intelligent force to guide you, to show you, to help you to *feel*, *see*, and *experience* more of this Subtle Reality. Then just relax and allow what arises in perception to be witnessed.

Releasing Dogma, or Fears which Prevent *Seeing*

Questioner: Maybe my "Christian" upbringing caused me to close-down perceptions of Subtle Energy.   Also, I am concerned about opening to harmful energies, when opening to Subtle Energy.

Darshan's reply: This "Christian" upbringing may indeed have contributed to shutting down or shifting your subtle perceptions out of focus.   But it is also a natural part of how we currently live in this very hypnotizing society, which with expert precision we constantly are being berated with all sorts of information, branding, and advertising, quite often without our best interest in mind.

When we realize that we cannot even believe everything that we ourselves think, then it is clear that we cannot believe everything that someone else thinks, believes, or lives according to.   And, we are also at this point of realization equipped with a key to go direct...   To perceive directly beyond the limits of these many contradicting concepts or ideas.

The Truth is that this Reality is vast and mysterious.   It is Infinite and unlimited and so it defies all description.

But this Infinity is also very simple. The direct Realization of this Truth can be pointed to with words, though it cannot be defined by them.

Many people think they know that God is omnipresent, omnipotent, omni powerful, and omniscient.... But few have directly contemplated this Truth. IF God is omnipresent, and omnipotent, Infinite and Unlimited, then there is nothing which is "outside" of or beyond That One. Every possible experience of being, and perception occurs within the Infinity of That One... This is the Power of Subtle Energy, which has also been "deified" as the Divine Mother Goddess, the very infinite power of God or all Infinity of Consciousness to experience all the infinite possibilities without limit.

So, this "Energy" is the very fabric of all we perceive... You are simply opening to See more of this Super Intelligent Force of Energy. Already what we perceive as form, identity, and knowledge is the movement of this field of Energy within Consciousness. If you feel you don't want to open to specific energies, you can always ask for the super intelligent force of energy, reiki, angels, (or whatever is a helpful resource to you) to guide and protect you while you open to perceive Subtle Energy.

This energy has also been recognized within the "Christian" system as the "holy spirit". But unfortunately, because of our own human ways of behaving we tend to misunderstand it when different terms are used. Thus, people from all different religions fight and perform terrible deeds to each other, even "Buddhists" and "Hindus" fight. This is all misunderstanding.

When we understand the simplicity of that God is the highest and only Truth, the indestructible Reality, and as such the source of the Light of Life and Consciousness in Every Being and Everything, then the natural "religion" is Love! Because then everywhere we look with the reverence of seeing the Supreme Being in Awesome Mystery of the Divine Play of all this!

In this way also, see that Divine Forces are always with you. And, though you can certainly be practical and not necessarily attune to, open to, or draw in "lower" unhelpful energies... Just don't even worry about it, let go of fear, Trust in your own inner strength, and the guidance of Divine forces in your life. When you fear something, or worry about it, you feed it energy or give it power. But these concepts, ideas, or phenomena of the world only hold as much power over you as you give them.

For now, you can breathe into, and open to specific energy that you know and trust. Apply the techniques and exercises the same but feel that you are homing in on just the energy of your choice. Then the keys remain to become as present as possible, and super aware. We are receiving this information at a subconscious level all the time anyways. So really, we are just becoming more aware of what we are already under the influence of, so we can be even more selective of what energies we nurture and allow to grow in our life.

Connecting with Guides & Guidance of Energy

Question: How to connect more, and hear guidance from my guides?

Darshan's Answer: Some of us receive guidance differently. Even when it is difficult to hear or talk to guides as you would converse with another person, one can still receive just as much or more information through other means.

The key is to become as present and clear as possible to be able to witness and receive this information. By clear Darshan means detaching from the thinking mind and drifting into stillness. Whether you are listening for the answer to a question from guides or becoming present to read the omens of the field, the more detached you are from the answer, and clear, then naturally the more clear you are to receive the info.

The Subtle Energy Mastery course Darshan is offering online is a simple system for becoming super present, clear, and still in order to interact with the Super Intelligent Force of Subtle Energy itself... Then we can receive guidance, and teachings directly from this Energy Field which is all pervasive, containing all vibration and thus all knowledge or all information. This Super Intelligent Energy is the very source and force of every energetic phenomena period...

In the deeper understanding of what is Energy or Power (Shakti) in the ancient esoteric lineages, this Energy is every single perceived phenomenon! All that is *seen*. Absolutely every movement that occurs in the equally infinite and all-pervasive field of Consciousness is this Super Intelligent Force of Energy. They, Consciousness and Energy, are "married"...

Who is *in* a body?

Many people think they are incarnated into a body. Like

you are a spirit in a body. Or you may tend to think you are Consciousness in a body.

But this is a bit of a mistake. A trick of the mind and perception where greater Awareness and the omni-presence of consciousness is lost. Because actually if you "look" closely you will notice that "your" consciousness is not in a body at all, and never was!

The body just as all phenomena, and appearances arises within the field of Consciousness. The body is within Consciousness, consciousness is not within the body. When you notice this, sinking deeper into consciousness you bring attention and awareness in on itself.

You then feel the expansion of consciousness, sometimes as if you are blown up way big like a giant balloon, and the body is really small within your expansive space. One way or the other just notice that consciousness is not stuck in a body, but simply the body is an experience arising within Consciousness. Then you can begin to expand Consciousness beyond old limited perception.

Consciousness is an all-pervasive phenomenon. A singular field. That is how certain Yogi's can know each if our thoughts intimately. We are clearly seen arising within the field of Consciousness. Merged with that omniscient

Consciousness, they can *see* every detail of this entire world and beyond within.

"Know thy Self", and *"The Truth will* [indeed] *set you free!"* The Truth is immortal freedom...

Japa (Repetition of Mantra)

Question: My mind is restless.   What to do?

Darshan's Answer: Many sages have said that in this age Nama Jap (repetition of the Mantra/Name of Divine) is the fastest, surest, easiest way to realize the Truth in this age... And, loving kindness put into action as selfless service.   The more you practice japa, naturally the more focused your mind, and energy will be, in all ways...

In response to a message that the writer had started practicing japa with the Mantra Om Namah Shivaaya as advised.

Darshan said: Excellent!   Remember that the Name is the Same as the Divine Presence!   It is only through the Grace that we even come to such an inclination to repeat the Holy Names...   How lucky we are!   This kind of "earnings" does not diminish even with death!

Om...

Mantra Diksha (Initiation)

Question: In the Babaji Manasa Yoga you give many mantras.   Do I need diksha to chant these mantras?

Darshan's Answer: Do not worry the mind too much about receiving or not having received Diksha.   Babaji is guiding your life, The Great Master will see to it that everything that is needed for your path will arrive in perfect Divine Timing.   The mantras given in the book are already a form of Diksha, they are coming with the intention of sharing in the energy generated by Darshan's literally millions of repetitions of mantra. The book is written with the Intention (Energy Anchored) for sharing Shaktipat Diksha. The book itself is also a manifestation of Babaji's Grace.

Babaji said once ""I have forgiven you of past transgressions. Now you must forgive yourself. You need only chant the Mahamantra and invoke my name to reach me."

"The teacher is here in the teachings. You have been initiated many lifetimes ago. Understand? Walk on the High Path and be a Beacon of Light for all sentient beings." -from the book: The Teachings of Babaji

The perpetuation of the idea that one must have contact with a Guru in physical form to receive diksha from is a misunderstanding of the omnipresence, inner meaning, and importance of the Guru. The Guru Tattva (Principle) is indeed a Force and Light without which That Perfection cannot be realized. Basically, this misunderstanding is a way of maintaining positions of religious power, where individuals claim that they are the holders of the True Knowledge, and thus that you must go through them to reach the Divine.

Actually, the Divine Perfection is the Absolute Reality, it is the Truth itself... It is everything else that appears to take away from that nature of our own Divine Power and Perfection which is false, temporary, or relative in comparison to That Infinite One. WE are all swimming in This Field of Illumined Awareness, our very own consciousness is sourced and rooted in That Infinite Illumined Awareness!

This light itself will provide all the energies and

"permissions" of Diksha. You can receive your Diksha Direct from the Most-High!

This one writing here now calls upon the Infinite all Pervasive Energy of Shakti. She who is the Form of the Energy which is transferred by all true Gurus in Shaktipat Diksha. We call this energy to Awaken within this one Reading. So that everything which is needed for Full Realization of the Supreme will be provided by this Limitless Energy (affectionately called Divine Mother - Shakti Kundalini).

Take time to center yourself through the breath, quiet the mind feeling anything that's there can just be set aside for a time.

Then call to Babaji and the Siddhars, expressing your deepest desire to connect with them.

Express your desire to receive the Dikshas or necessary energies to fully energize your practice and speed you along The Way.

Know that this Energy is already there and working from the Subtle Dimensions of your Being.

Take a meditative period to consciously connect with this guidance and acknowledge that you are receiving everything that is needed for your pathway.

At this time with the multitudes of bodies on earth and people with misleading and devious intentions acting out in ignorance of the nature of Self/God, it sometimes can be hard to find a good Representative of the Guru in a body... The Siddhars knowing this are working all the more to ensure that those links are provided in other ways when they are needed. If it will truly be beneficial for you to have a Bodily Guru one will be provided. You will find them and recognize the Guru when the time is right! But with or without, know that the Siddhars are with you and guiding, feel that you have everything and all the tools at your disposal.

If you say a mantra 125,000 times (on average) that mantra will indeed activate to a strength in your Heart chakra and energy field, to the point that YOU could give someone Diksha in that Mantra while passing special energy of the mantra to help.

There are even stories from the ancient scriptures of someone hearing part of the Vaak Bija mantra- AIM from a pig and repeating this sound (only part of the full mantra) with devotion. The Goddess Saraswati appeared and granted boons to the mispronouncing reciter!

So, don't worry the mind too much about these things. It is clear to this one writing that Maha Avatar Babaji is guiding you based on your experiences with Him. That One's Power and Guidance does not fail! That omnipresent Babaji provides the Highest of Dikshas. Every time you take His Name, He hears you and is with you. You may or may not be able to hear Him and See His Presence there with you (until you become more accustomed to noticing the Subtle) but Babaji is certainly able to hear you.

It is just one of the tricks of the mind to find ways that it needs to seek outside of itself. This way the tyrant continues its perch and position. When we just let go of everything in the mind for a time and just let the mind fold in on itself, then we can see that the contents of mind whatever they may be have just been waves on the surface of an Infinite Ocean of Consciousness. Beneath these surface waves of thoughts, the Illumined All Pervasive Field of Awareness - SambaSadaShiva is ever present.

Diksha Continued & Babaji Light Body Meditation

Questioner Again: I feel strong energy from Babaji and the Siddhar but I don't really know what to do during sadhana. I have already chanted many mantras however these mantras are different from the ones that you give in the Babaji's Manasa Yoga book. Could you tell me more about Babaji Sadhana to reach the higher state of reality and being? The light body/rainbow body?

Darshan's Answer: You can continue to work with the mantras which you have already generated a connection with.

If you have received mantra diksha from a Great Saint like Amma, then this mantra practice should definitely be kept up, and this kind of Mantra Diksha does indeed have special power because of Amma's Power. The mantra is specific to the receiver's needs, and because of the power of the Guru manifest through Her, the mantra diksha Amma gives is a promise. By following instructions and chanting the mantra Realization is guaranteed...

If you feel drawn to work with any of the mantras from the book, feel free to do so without any doubt that they are working. Devotion is the ultimate key and pin by which all mantras and Deities are bound. It is not necessary to learn all the mantras from the book. Or repeat them all, the point of including them in the text was just provide some practical options for ways of proceeding with sadhana. Even one syllable of the Great Wisdom of the Sages and Seers repeated with faith and firm determination is enough!

Sadhana is becoming efficient with one's focus, energy, and activity. When one can become aware enough to know truly what it is that they want, one can then start to effectively manage and channel their energy, focus, and activity towards that goal. When it comes to the realization of the Ultimate, That Pure Awareness can only be witnessed, experienced and known by That Pure Awareness itself. Because everything that is and is not is *seen* by means of That Light of Awareness. Thus, everything *seen* is like a reflection in the medium of That Infinite Field of Awareness, and not the Wholeness of Awareness Itself...

Sadhana then in this case is not the cause of That Illumined Awareness which is itself the primary cause and medium within which all causes are seen. The Grace of the Light of Awareness is the cause of Sadhana. For the True Sadhak who will settle for nothing less than the Infinite Awareness, sadhana is removing all obstacles of relative perception to reveal that Absolute Essence of the Illumined Being.

In this way shift the way that you do your mantras and other practices so that the focus is on the Ideal itself, rather than working towards a goal, with every repetition affirm/Invoke here now the Absolute Reality of Divine Nature.

Practices of sadhana are very simple, it's just the repetition or continuous application that is the key. Mind is an infinite field of possibilities as to what and how the stories of perception can be. Repeatedly we must bring the state of mind away from complexity, division, and "figuring it out" and back to rest in its own nature of that infinite potential of Being.

Turning the body to light results from integration or surrender to the Absolute Reality (Infinite Power and Potential) at all levels of being all the way into the cells of the Body. If Absolute Reality is Immortal Limitless Light, then realizing this at a cellular level the cells are this Infinite Light as well...no? Love is also a requirement for full Light Body activation, for it Is the Realization of the Truth of All Life as One.

Darshan feels that you already know more about sadhana practice than you may think. But this is just the nature of mind, it can distract itself into infinity by its infinite potential of perceptions. Just dive down into the depths of mind. Turn seeking within as to who is thinking? Who is listening or believes the story portrayed by thoughts? Where do the thoughts originate? Turn awareness to the field of awareness itself. Or watch the field of awareness dancing with energy (all that is witnessed within awareness are movements of energy). Step back as a pure witness uninvolved with what is *seen*.

Turn focus with sharpening intensity through practice on Babaji and His Realized State. All that is and is not, everything and nothing is within your Field of Awareness and Energy. Focusing on Babaji and the Siddhas you are attuning to their station and states of mind within your own awareness. They exist merged with subtle levels of your being. Learn to just let the thoughts be and shift focus to these subtle places in your being and you feel their Power. This Power is guiding you from within.

This Power of the concentrated Intent of Enlightened Beings is vastly more powerful than the briefly rising and falling relative mind states. Focus on That Enlightened Intention. Let go of any confusion, doubt, or feeling of not having the required tools.

Breathe this focus of the Absolute Perfection (Babaji)

into the cells of the body. Imagine that the cells are breathing in Immortal Light - the Truth - Absolute Reality, and breathing out all the relative, limited, or dense.

If you sit for even just 15-20 minutes per day consciously breathing the Grace and Light of Babaji into the Cells, while breathing out any apparent obstacles, there will be profound results. At least twice per day would be recommended, and to repeat mantra mentally or aloud as often as possible. Just these two practiced with consistency would be profound and efficient sadhana.

Sleep and Dream Yoga, and Sahaja (Natural) Meditation

In response to an email asking Darshan to share any advice about practices while sleeping, dream yoga, and Sahaja (natural, surrender, or effortless meditation)

Darshan's reply: Yes, sahaja is natural, in the Avadhuta Gita Dattatreya uses sahajamrtam (translated to the nectar of naturalness) "For the destruction of the terrible poisonous universe, which produces the unconsciousness of delusion, there is but one infallible remedy-the nectar of naturalness." - Swami Ashokananda translation of Avadhuta Gita

Sahaja Meditation is also called surrender meditation. It involves just sitting, without making efforts of concentration of contemplation. Simply allowing the Divine Consciousness itself to direct the attention, and experience of meditation. It can also mean becoming just the pure witness or observer, not identifying with whatever appears in Awareness. Not trying to push away, cling to or manipulate an appearance within mind. A perfect example of "sahaja meditation" is when we went to have a silent sitting meditation with a Self-Realized Swamiji in Rishikesh India, he said as we sat for meditation before beginning "don't do anything [with/in the mind] just relax...".

Sahaja Samadhi is said to be "higher" than nirvikalpa samadhi (sitting with eyes closed and the senses completely withdrawn, and the object of concentration dissolved...), where one functions naturally in daily life, while always remaining in a state of samadhi...

I do highly recommend yoga while sleeping and dreaming... The simplest is to engage in japa while falling asleep and training the mind to repeat japa through the night, so any time you wake up you find yourself with the mantra, and in the morning the same. While travelling in India the last time, I had stopped briefly in Hardwar while travelling from the south back to "home" village Haidakhan. While there I took refuge (slept for a few days) under a tree that was kept by "Monkey Baba" a beautiful sadhu. One night when I got up to urinate, I noticed one of the other baba's sleeping under the tree was engaged in japa. It's almost funny the way it sounded, because you could tell from his voice that he was clearly deep asleep... But a deep slow "om namoh narayan" was repeated audibly again and again from his lips while he slept...

A way to go lucid, is to hold (maintain) awareness as everything falls asleep. Just drop into the meditative states as you would while awake, you are already then accessing the same brainwave states as in sleep and dream. Then just hold the awareness, keep awareness awake while you allow the body and conscious mind to fall asleep...

A Technique Learned in a Dream

In response to a message where the sender had a

dream where Darshan Baba told them to do a new breathing technique (Pranayama) and demonstrated the movement of the energy with a handheld model. Thus, they reached out to get clarification about the technique.

Darshan replied: Not consciously sure of the answer currently in this "waking" state. But the enquiry came just when we were recently discussing getting back to practicing during the dream state more deeply, with "lucid dreaming" practices... The message further inspires the idea of doing group dream work. Where we can form a group to facilitate and support each other along in increasing lucidity and practical application of the dream state.

As we all increase our lucidity and "exercise our dreaming mind" we can meet as a group in the dream state and together explore new states of Awareness, visit sacred realms such as siddha lok, and consult with perfected masters...

It feels that the answer is with you. As you recall the instruction, Feel into the technique as it is being relayed. What does it feel like in your energy body, as Darshan shows the object to demonstrate? Trust, and follow your intuition. Allow yourself to be clear, and connect deeply into the information you are carrying within the "mind/body" energy field from the dream. Allow yourself to relax and breathe into this space of direct knowing, to allow the technique to occur under the guidance of super intelligence, while dropping having to figure it out or "know" logically...

There is no limit to infinity. "New" technologies can and will emerge. We have been conditioned into discrediting of our own clear direct and intuitive connection to Infinity... But this infinity always has been and will always be within you. More and more trust in your own direct connection, guidance from, and "embodiment" of the Infinite!

Don't Attach to the Coming and Going of Yogic Experiences

Question: Upset that a mala just broke, and wondering if it is good or bad? Also, though I am more committed to my pathway of Sadhana and more disciplined, I am not having as many visions, feeling energy etc. while meditating as used to.

Darshan's reply: Mala breaking is generally considered an auspicious omen... There have been times when this body somehow could not keep any malas together for weeks, every new mala bought broke within a couple of days!   This body was nearly constantly engaged in japa at the time, so they were getting heavy use. But still, it was uncanny how they just kept coming apart right away.

Yogic experiences arise and fall naturally as do all movements of cognition within the infinite medium of Consciousness with limitless Power to experience Being. As such, grasping for such experiences or wondering where they have gone can simply make it less open for such experiences to again naturally arise.   When you understand or intuit what is the "Supreme Practice" then always return to That.   Do not be fooled by tendency of mind to waver, wander, and grasp for this and that.

Remember that: "Yoga chitta vrtti nirodha." Yoga happens when mental gymnastics stop, or no longer entrap focus.   Everything, am "I doing this right, which is higher or lower, is it working, I am meditating, whatever"... These are all the waves, the vritti.   Focus beyond!

Allow Sakti to work, and the Super Intelligent Force of creation certainly will.   The Divine Energy is already at work in your life.   So, bring about more feeling of an open state where you can ALLOW the energy to continue to guide these experiences.   A subtle inner shift brings about perception of your efforts to become less of "your" effort and more surrender to the Divine Inherent Truth which is unraveling your pathway before you.

Every time you say the Name it is this Divine Presence and Grace.   Krishna said He is where His Names are being kept with devotion... His Name is God.

So, look directly within and *see* if you can find who is really "saying" the mantra or doing "your" japa. Is it you?

Or, if you consider it carefully, can you really say that YOU have EVER done anything at all...?

"I" mean, after all, or before it all,

WHO ARE YOU???   REALLY...?

Question: I had a spontaneous Kundalini Awakening experience over 22 years ago while performing pranayama.   It left with a sensitivity that was nearly frying the nervous system.   Have had these experiences a handful of times over the years since then.   A couple years ago I took shaktipat from a few different in person and distant facilitators.   Now I have the obvious effects of the shaktipat as spontaneous kriyas, laughing, crying, or body shaking etc.   But I don't get the flashes of illumination that came with my previous awakening experiences. Before I was practicing Raja Yoga, and now since having received Shaktipat it is like Ma Shakti is controlling me, and I am not sure that I like it, or that I am progressing. It feels like I have transgressed, and I still have this yearning that is so intense, to be back in that illumination.

Darshan's Answer: The simple answer to your question is surrender... Align your burning intensity of yearning for this illumination with Trust, Faith, and Patience.

Ultimately, as you describe, your spontaneous illumination experience came with an "Awakening of Kundalini"... So, you will see that there is a "slight of hand" division being reflected by your mind which is interrupting your progress. For you are yearning with an intensity for Shakti (Kundalini) to Awaken in you, yet on the other hand your mind feels as if you cannot trust Shakti to be in control.

However, you can see that She (Shakti) is already in control... And, always had been, even before you had shaktipat dikshas. This subtle force is ALL form Svarupini, the power, vibration, and medium of every single experience which arises within the medium of Infinite Consciousness (Siva). She - Shakti - Kundalini - Maha Maya, is the limitless Power of this Infinite Self to experience Being.

You can be certain that "progress" IS occurring, which the spontaneous kriyas are a part of. This Super-Intelligent force knows with perfection and certainty what and where needs to be unlocked in the "body" and energy-field. So, Sakti is performing Maha Yoga for you, or kriya yog, siddha yog, sahaja yog...

IF it helps to bring a feeling of greater direction/progress, alignment, etc. you can still practice your previous techniques of Raja Yoga. But also take time to Allow Super-Intelligent Sakti to work for you.

You will remember that the first Illumination experience you felt like the new Cosmic level of Sakti/Energy and the INCREDIBLE amount of additional information which this includes was near to frying the nervous system and bringing the mind to the edge of insanity. Now Kundalini Sakti, Jagad Ambe Maa is making the system ready for sustainable integration of increased Energetic Capacity.

Also allow the practice itself to be the Realization of the Supreme Teaching. In other words, don't be attached to this outcome of the Yogic Experience, but simply surrender into full presence of the moment. Be Aware, Alert, and fully present with the breath, Sakti (Pure

Power), and Siva (Infinite Consciousness). Darshan can resonate with and understand your position, as have also gone through periods of difficulty in attaining certain yogic experiences from the past, simply because of attachment to or expectation for them.

But we can remember these experiences are in the past and gone, a dream... A distraction from noticing That Same Infinity is right here Now at All times. The Truth always remains the Truth. It has gone nowhere, That Illumination in which all time and space arises, never goes anywhere.

Ultimately there is only one Giver of Shaktipat, Shakti Herself. Trust in That and you can burn through all obstacles.

Sudden Unusual Experience, like "Altered" States

Question: Have you ever experienced a spontaneous trip [psychedelic like experience]? Am three days into one, and a little worried...

Darshan's Answer: Just breathe... No matter what it is. It's just energy!   Trust in the very Force of Life living Life! And, don't worry...   Direct your ideas of identity to the feet, and guiding hand of Divinity.

You will be fine.   God/dess cannot fail.   our ideas of self or ego are always failing.   But the Divine One, source of life, all Awareness, and the medium of All Perceptions, cannot fail!

If there is any resistance anxiety fear etc. look to *see* directly where it is coming from, and why, not to think about it but look directly to See.   Same with any intense medicine experience (traditional "power plant" psychedelics used by shamans, such as Ayahuasca, Psilocybe Mushrooms, Peyote, etc.)   Contemplate looking directly to *see* where any tension is coming from and why...   Rather than focusing on and feeding the surface waves of the appearance of this tension of anxiety, look for the root, the source, and the "experiencer" of these.   And, remember to just breathe, every experience will pass or change in time.

Questioner again in a later message: My spontaneous trip has dramatically improved my life.   ...specifically, if you need a question to focus on: what the heck is god doing in that space?   ...not just me, many people have found "god" while tripping.   The space I refer to is the psychedelic state...   ...I worry there is too much power there...

Darshan's reply: Every space is within God (Totality/Wholeness of Omniscient Being. All/Omnipresent Consciousness) ...

Siva is pure all-pervasive Awareness/Consciousness. All Consciousness.   All ONE field of Consciousness...   All of the Universe appears within That.   Shakti is Energy/Maya All appearances.   Everything that is seen including perceived within, is that Power (Shakti). She/Shakti is called Svarupini-all form, vagishvari-all vibration. Siva is the Seer, the Self of All. Shakti the Power of the Self to experience Being, manifesting within That Infinite Field of Awareness all the Infinite phenomena of appearances/experiences!

Spontaneous Kundalini Kriyas

In response to a message seeking guidance about suddenly waking up one day with the body doing Yoga

Sadhana postures, movements etc. spontaneously, without any effort.

Darshan's response: You can look up, automatic kundalini kriyas, or spontaneous kriyas... It is associated with kundalini waking up in the body. And, by the direction of this Super Intelligence of Shakti (Energy) kriyas (or yoga techniques) spontaneously occurring to release samskaras, or energy blockages.

So basically, people will practice all these different techniques by their own efforts to attain yogic experiences, attainments, or realizations. But, when what is happening to you occurs, the actions are being directed by the Super Intelligence of Kundalini Shakti which can be far superior to our own efforts... Because this Super Intelligent form of and source of all Energy knows exactly how to work or direct the kriyas.

Connect more deeply to Shakti as Divine Mother to allow you to surrender into greater trust, faith, and patience in the process. So that if you can view it as a gift of the Grace from the Goddess, then it can be related to as a blessing in gratitude, rather than just a strange experience.

Questioner Again: What goddess?! Is there such a thing?

Darshan's reply: It is just a way of relating to the Energy moving your body to relate with the experience in a way that it can be "familiar".   To recognize and trust in the Super Intelligence of the Energy.   If it doesn't work for you to consider the Energy moving your body spontaneously as "the Goddess", forget it... But, try to find a way to trust the process.   So, it doesn't seem like a struggle, with the mind, or appearance of a "personal" identity fighting the experience.

You can also ask this Energy to take it easy, be more gentle, or leave you alone...   But, it is an incredibly fortunate opportunity.   Which has naturally occurred. So, by the Omniscient Intelligence of the Divine Energy, one and the same in all, it had been determined beneficial to you, that you are ready, and can integrate this.   If you can just leave your thinking mind out of it, to allow the process to be.   It requires finding a way to trust that it is a helpful thing to your life.

You don't have to think of it as "God" if it's not helpful to you.   "God" is just a word and a concept.   But Consciousness and Energy are indisputable

Questioner again: So, it seems, I'm a puppet.

Darshan's reply: The ego is like a puppet, you are not the thinking mind (ego).   You are indestructible

Consciousness which is itself the puppet master. But we have forgotten who we really are, and so are living in the experience of something no more significant than a form of thought which can come and go. By realizing that every idea of ourselves is a thought perceived we can settle deeper into our Reality of Being by searching for the perceiver itself.

One suggestion would be that you can do that in relation to the "strange" occurrences of the body performing yoga all by itself. As any resistance, discomfort, etc. arises in the mind about what is happening, instead of feeding and believing these perceptions, inquire directly with your attention as to from where do these perceptions arise. Such as, who or what is causing this? Who resists it? Who is afraid? Who do you take yourself to be? A thought which can change from one view to the next in an instant?

You are letting your mind trick you. You will have to let go of all your ideas of the world and your "self" even to be open to the possibilities of solutions and assistance. Otherwise you are closing yourself off to continue to be a servant of your own mind. When the mind is meant to serve you.

Why not just be free? You came into the world naked, without a name, or all these concepts about life... How can it be said that it should be like this and not like that or any way at all, rather than just as it's happening. You could connect to and ask for help from Tapasyogi Nandhi. Or one of his Teachers Annai Siddhar Raju Kumar Swami, who is a master of Kundalini attainment. You could also connect to Maha Sambodhi Dharma Sangha Guru and His direct guidance in/through the heart.

In response to various chatter, or complaints about the experience and circumstances. Darshan said: All these things you are mentioning are just from your mind. You need to distinguish between what is just noise the mind is making, and ego. And, who really are you?

Mind like body, just appears within you [Consciousness]. It is a bad habit we "modern" humans have to identify ourselves with these appearances.

May it all work out beautifully for you. You are very lucky. Your mind is just fighting to maintain its position as king rather than servant... Realizing that something other than your thinking mind or who you take yourself to be is in charge of this whole thing. Try asking that force which appears to be in charge, for help to understand and integrate this. Or, to guide you wherever or to whoever can help.

Questioner again: So, I'm possessed? Is it Kundalini or

possession?

Darshan's answer: Don't be confused. You yourself are directing all this, from a level beyond the "personally" identified mind, from Super Consciousness/Intelligence. You are just living in a pocket of thought which feels as if it is a puppet. Because the thoughts are not in control of the thinker. Just don't identify with/as the thoughts.

Questioner again replying with specific details about the incredible (and rare) nature of their experience, and the fear or worry about it due to the unique nature of this incredible experience and lack of resources to guide about or understand this phenomenon of Real Kundalini Awakening.

Darshan replied with a set of pictures of Powerful Siddha Masters who we have Great Faith in. And, who are omnipresent with their Grace and Power to support and guide us. Darshan said: Be at Peace.

Questioner again: The pictures of the masters link me to them?

Darshan's answer: The picture link to their blessings and support... You are not alone. We are all in this together. And the super intelligent energy of the Life force within your body is itself directing the body in yoga perfectly. The only issue is the ego mind is fighting with or unwilling to surrender in trust of the process.   Which is also natural.

Questioner talking about ego, and wisely expressing the desire for a living Guru who understood exactly the process they were going through to guide them.

Darshan's reply: "Ego" (identification) is a natural function in mind.   Just learn to relax back from it and distinguish between what is just noise in the mind, and what is really you.   Gain the power to choose where your attention and identity is placed...   If you know the difference, then don't give yourself up to what you are not.

Darshan suggested and sent links to some Siddhas, and Masters, who were of a level of genuine attainment to be able to guide the questioner.   Darshan said: Sorry to say, a good and genuine Guru qualified to guide you in the level of your experience is rare and hard to find.   But this heart has Great Faith in the Energy working in your Life to guide you right to where you need to be.   Sorry it's not always pink and fluffy for the ego.   And, can even mean life seeming to fall apart.   But if you can make it through the process.   It will guaranteed be beneficial in your overall quality of life.

Questioner asking why a specific Guru or his followers

would not let them stay at the ashram/community, and they were told to leave.

Darshan's answer: Don't know why about [Guru's name). He maybe is just not for you. You may have a very old relationship with another very powerful Guru who you will find. Just try to relax and trust in the Super Intelligence of the Universe and very Life Force to guide you wherever or to whoever you need to go. Life is living Life itself, the thought of "me" is not the source or doer of this Life.

Questioner again: Does this happen often to people? Is it normal to live with it [Kundalini Shakti] dancing you [moving body in spontaneous kriyas] all the time? Do other people do this like this?

Darshan's answer: No. This is very rare. You are very lucky. Some would consider it a high attainment in Yoga. Because the ego can perform hardcore Sadhana for ages and get nowhere. But when the "efforts" of yoga are coming from the Divine Energy itself, then it is pretty sure success by the Super Intelligence of yoga itself. Be blessed with Peace and Greater Ease in your Process Divine One. May all the guidance you are seeking arrive swiftly.

Questioner again: My entire frustration is that the

books and mediators say be still and watch this or that... But being still makes me dance. So, am I doing it wrong; should I try and be still or trust it and let it happen?

Darshan's answer: Just trust... allow your mind to rest and the body to dance if it wants.

Darshan's commentary for this book: The one who sent this enquiry seeking guidance, had a very rare experience of spontaneous awakening of ongoing active Kundalini Shakti after a prayer.   The Shakti had awakened to an uncomfortable level without preparation, and without proper guidance, though the questioner had been seeking such guidance since the awakening.   The nature of their experience was very intense with the body being nearly constantly moved by itself in "spontaneous kundalini kriyas".   Spontaneous kundalini kriyas occur when the body is moved by the Kundalini Shakti (Energy) itself without one's own apparent efforts, making yoga postures, and movements all by itself.

This also became very difficult for them due to a lack of understanding of what was happening to the questioner by family and friends around them, making it look "strange" or "crazy" to the onlookers.   They were not by any means just "complaining".   They had very real and intense experiences occurring without any foreknowledge to understand what was happening.   And, the difficulty with lack of support from a good community or Teacher (Guru) made their life seem to fall apart, with the loss of many things dear to them.

We need more Awareness of these kinds of occurrences, and a general attitude of non-judgement and loving support of our fellow humans no matter how unfamiliar or strange it may seem to us whatever may be happening in another's life. We don't want to shut out or judge someone because they have entered new territory of life which seems "crazy" to our idea of life and the world.

The Siddha Subtle Energy Medicine & Shaktipat empowerment facilitated/channeled by Darshan Baba is gentle. The Energy is transmitted and activated by and under the Guidance of the Super Intelligent force of All Energy itself. Thus no one has ever reported such an uncomfortable experience of Kundalini Shakti awakening. Though it can also be very powerful as one receiver said "it felt like being hit with a lightning bolt", it should never move faster than one is capable of handling, mentally, physiologically, and energetically. On the contrary, if one had such an uncomfortable or unbalanced spontaneous Shakti awakening, or similar experience with a Shaktipat that left one without the proper guidance, the Siddha Subtle Energy Medicine and Shaktipat Empowerment from Darshan should help to balance out and ease the awakening in an integrateable way.

This direct connection with all Perfected Masters combined and Guru Tattva (principle of the guiding light of Awakening) facilitated by the Siddha Energy Medicine and Shaktipat, will help to guide the receiver synchronistically. To whatever resources and experiences "internally" or "externally" that will bring about full awakening in an integrated and balanced way. This is facilitated by the Super Intelligence of the Grace of Pure Energy (Shakti), the Perfected Masters (Siddha), guiding Light of Self-Realized Being (Guru), and the very Way (Marga) of Harmony (Dharma). The marga or pathway exists like an Energetic edifice of its own within the Infinity of Being and Consciousness. Dharma as well, is already occurring within the Super Intelligence of the Wholeness of Omniscient Being. Whether we know these things intellectually or not. They are a Power of their own, which we can align with and benefit from.

The methods of Sadhana, the Shaktipat, Subtle Energy training, courses, books, guidance etc. offered by Darshan are all about discovering and exercising one's ability to directly align with and receive this presence and guidance of the Super Intelligence of Infinity itself. This is the only infallible way, attaining your own Direct Connection to the Way (Marga), the Guiding Light of Awakening (Guru), the Harmony of the Whole (Dharma) and Direct *Seeing* power.

Then you cannot be deceived or misled, even by your own mind or ego. When you can *See* with the direct connection of Super Intelligence, it becomes clear what is and what is not.

Self-Realization

Question: I am writing to you with one hope, one prayer, can you please help me realize myself? Is this Grace possible? My only aim in life is to realize my true Self, to find the answers to the question, Who Am I?

Darshan's Answer: If you truly have only one aim, to realize the Self then it shall be so. With that aim and Sankalpa shakti (firm determination) look to see from where do thoughts emerge, who listens, who responds, who believes the thoughts?

Everything that is seen (all perception) is in a state of constant motion and change. Thus, the ancient instructions of the Vedic Seers is a simple "not this, not this" to all that is Seen. As Mooji would say contemplate on "can the Seer of all this itself be Seen?"

Dattatreya said " Always not this, not this to both the formless and the formed, only the Absolute (Sivah) exists, transcending difference, and non-difference." -Swami Ashokananda translation of the Avadhuta Gita

Look to within for a State of Being which has always been the same, unchanging and constant. Imagine everything you perceive, your identity, comprehension of the world and knowledge, everything burning in the Fire of Truth, with only the indestructible Immortal Truth of the Self to remain...

Darshan's Commentary for this book: Many times, we may think that we really want only Self-Realization, but in fact our energy is not completely aimed at only this one goal.   We think it is the case, but if we look mindfully at our life and state of mind, we may find that actually we are still invested in various desires, and activities towards other goals or results.   When we really truly have only this one desire alone for Self-Realization, and the Firm-Determination for this then we will certainly have that realization shortly...

Why wouldn't it be so? The Essential Truth of Being is already the Reality of who we are.   It is only because we are dreaming many other ideas, identity, or pursuits over that One unmovable nature that we miss "What Is" Naturally.   As soon as we are really willing to give up what is not, for what is, then Ultimate Being will only be.

In reply to an email with updates from one of our recipients of Shaktipat on their sadhana for Self-Realization.

Darshan's Answer: The "I" is more real than the appearances of "body" and "mind".   But the "I" has most often been mis-identified as the body, mind, and imagined features of one's "identity" (such as name, family, parents, culture etc.).   The feeling of "I" or the Self is One and is the same in All.   Thus "i" (Darshan Baba) engaged in a sadhana of not using the words I or me in relation to this body or mind.   Because I am not the body or mind, and they are not "mine".   They simply appear spontaneously within the infinite medium of the Self as expression of the Infinite Possibility to experience Being.

Understand this body and mind do not belong to a limited idea of "me" who was born, but they belong to the One, the Absolute Reality- God/dess. This I is appearing in all bodies, and none of them.   So how can that One speak from a limited form and say this substance which has no lasting reality is "I" or "me"?   It is like forgetting everything accept the hand and from here speaking of "I" and mine without realizing that the hand belongs to the body and is but a small piece.

The Truth is that the Self is already of the Nature of Moksha - Pure Freedom...   Sakti brought by the shaktipat is burning away the clusters of energy and thought forms that have become stuck in ignorance of our True identity. This True Identity which has no identity, is the source and medium of all possibilities of experience in Being...   And, even this appearance of identity, name, and form is just the expression of the limitless possibilities of the Infinite Being.

In this way shift the fire of aspiration/sadhana just ever so slightly, to that you are clearly burning away that which is not real... (Instead of the burning desire for Union, this fire is Burning as the very Presence of Union growing in Intensity removing all unreality of division). The Union of the Absolute IS ABSOLUTE, that Infinity is the Only Reality, none of this can be without that Pure Consciousness in Union with Infinite Power/Potential/Energy (SambaSadaShiv), and all witnessed experience arises within That Medium.

Babaji's Promise of Moksha

Babaji said that whoever even hears of Haidakhan Vishwa Mahadham will have moksha. As well as whoever goes there, bathes in the Gautami Ganga river, drinks from the Ram Dhara Spring, visits the Maha Moksha Dhuni, etc.

Through effort of Kriya it takes incredible focus and discipline. Whereas the Super Intelligent Sakti can carry information and experience beyond the limits of action, reason, and words at lightning rapid speed. This Shakti (Energy) is even working beyond the dimensions of time.

Everything witnessed is composed and informed by Sakti/Energy. For every atom or particle of apparent "matter" there are over a Billion bits of Information as Energy/Sakti ($E=mc2$). Thus, the Super Intelligent Sakti carries incredible amounts of information, and can indeed blaze through the sadhak as the Sakti-Energy/Gyan-Knowledge of Liberation.

Furthermore, by the limitless Power (Shakti) of the Maha Siddha Yogi's such as Mahamunindra Maharaj the promise of Moksha is SURE...

The Maha Siddha Babaji's Promise of Moksha is more

durable than words set in stone. The Sakti of a Maha Siddha's Promise is more Real than any doubts or limitations of the "practitioner". Without Sakti (The Divine Energy) there is no phenomena seen whatsoever.

Anyone who Completely Surrenders to the Power (Shakti) of Babaji's Promise of Moksha will certainly be Liberated by the unfailing Divine Energy/Maha Shakti. This Maha Maya Shakti is the Source and Form of All Phenomena and thus is more Real than all these appearances. As it says in the Chandi Path/Durga Sapta Shati - That Energy/Shakti is the form of knowledge AND ignorance, harmony and lack of harmony, and All the Infinite Possibilities of Pure Consciousness (Siva) to experience Being. The Divine Energy is the very medium of the ever-Expanding Infinity.

Every time you say the Name of Babaji, He hears you... Concentrate on Him. He is as Alive as ever, and always near! Just think of Him. Naturally everything else falls into place.

The mind gets busy, bring it back to Him. This is the Simplicity.

Spiritual Powers

Question: Are there any people in the world with Real Spiritual Powers?

Darshan's reply: "Spiritual" Power is not different than the very Life Force. The Light of Awareness and its Infinite Power to Experience Being... Therefore, all beings alive have "Real Spiritual Power", or in other words are only alive because of their Real "Spiritual" Power. When this Power wanes and drains due to lack of compassion or Understanding of the Infinite All Pervasive Nature of Being then naturally the force of Life leaves from the body.

Question about the book "Cosmic Consciousness and Healing with the Quantum Field"

Question: I noticed that the Moksha Gyan Books have a very strong quality of transmission... I have been very reluctant about taking up practices that come with qualities of transmission unknown to me.   I am skeptical of artificially installing a healing gift that was not developed by natural sadhana. When I read about calling on a divine healing-team I again was reluctant. Many people channel astral beings and one cannot be sure if the information from astral beings is always valid. Can you provide more information about the origin of this practice, and about the energy qualities these books are working with?

Darshan's Answer: Happy to answer your question, as best as this mind is able, do forgive writing style, as this body has been practicing a sadhana of eliminating use of the words I, me, mine and the like for over a year now... [April 2012]

The Level of Reality which these transmissions originate from is not something which is outside of yourself. This mind takes your hesitation for external "artificial programing" of your energy field to be a sincerity for true sadhana practice.

The nature of these transmissions and attunements being of the Primordial Essence of Pure Energy (with infinite possibilities) in Ecstatic marriage with All Pervasive Awareness - there is no limit to the ways they can manifest. This is something of the Divine Nature which is the source and Light of All Life manifesting throughout all levels of That One Infinite Being. The Intention of the book is that these energies bring forth only possibilities which are in harmony with each one's particular pathway. The point is to open to this dimension of Reality which is an infinite field of Pure Energy. Then use from those infinite resources whatever will benefit one's greater empowerment, awareness, and awakening.

True sadhana is removing obstacles to Yoga, or experience of Total Union - the "individual" consciousness dissolving into Total experience of that Primordial Awareness (Siva) and Limitless Energy (Shakti). Sadhana then is not the cause of this Total Awareness of Yoga, as it is by this Primordial Power and Awareness that all that is and is not is caused and witnessed. So, in this way all developments of sadhana, instructions, and empowerments/transmissions which appear on the gross level of reality are actually first caused from this First Light of Awareness which is the cause of awakening. This is synonymous with the Force of Grace! The Guru - the illumined being within, and all manifestations of the Guru in bodies - certainly wants this Awakening of Love (All Life as One), for All of Life.

Whatever "tricks" of gross manifestation which are necessary or helpful to turn the mind towards its own nature, will manifest by the Force of that Grace of Awakening. The omnipresent Light of Awareness is the very source of all consciousness. As has been said by the

Illumined Ones repeatedly - our own nature is Enlightenment. Sadhana is removing coverings to witness this Absolute Truth of Being.

In this way receiving transmissions for these energies to flow is not an artificial installation of healing gift. It is Sadhana to accept one's Divine Nature and All the Gifts that come with That. These energies do indeed cause changes in the energy field, but they cannot and will not work in ways that you are not open and accepting of them to work.

The Divine Being with Limitless Power would give us all immense gifts. All of this universe is a product of that infinity, with infinite other dimensions (layered simultaneously) of possibilities in different modes of experience. In this way incredibly diverse are the ways of empowering us which are manifest.

In Reiki attunements for example, a whole group could be attuned, but how that gift of energy is utilized will be different among the "individuals". Some will practice with this energy with great faith and become great healers. Others might just move onto the next weekend workshop never really learning or integrating anything.

The necessity for sadhana in order to accept and utilize these gifts is still present. In fact, if in the mode of sadhana one attains constant one-pointed concentration on the life force (Reiki), who's to say the body won't turn to light?   But we don't see everyone who is getting reiki attunements turning to light...

Regarding the Healing Team: You are correct that all sorts of information and entities can be floating through the Astral Field and other dimensions of awareness... Indeed, don't accept any nonsense, but connect only with helpful beings and resources.   Your Healing Team (whether you are aware of it or not) involves only symbols, figures, deities, Awareness, or Energies that serve your personal pathway.   It could be one Master who embodies All useful resources, of even just the Primordial All-Pervasive Awareness itself appearing as personified or deified form for our understanding/relating.

The point of these books is to offer tools for resources in greater well-being and awakening.   The only magic pill is [surrender to] That One Primordial Light of All-pervasive Awareness with Limitless Power...   That Infinite Energy is constantly offering up all of the possibilities of Maha Maya. That Infinite One Alone Exists.   All that is Witnessed cannot be anyway separate from That Awareness and Power.   That Power is your own Nature.   It is our Awareness.   Nothing is more real than That Consciousness with Infinite Power to Experience Being. Take and utilize whatever tools re-empower awareness with the Infinite Peace and Possibilities of the Divine Play of That One Infinite Field of Awareness. In the end none of the tools are real and That One Alone is... Love (All Life as One)!

When Other's Won't Listen

Question: How does this body point others to the truth when no one will listen because of the way society has told them this body should act because of its age? They say this body knows nothing because it is 16. When this mind tries to express that age means nothing, they turn away from the truth this body is trying to impart.

Darshan's Answer: This is an interesting point indeed, and unfortunately you cannot change others minds or conditioning, all you can do is commit yourself ever greater to the pathway of living this Truth, because though people may not be able to hear you words, your actions in time will speak even louder than words...

For example, the Nepali Param Atma Avatar they were calling the Buddha Boy, went and sat under the Tree at age of 16 sitting in unbroken meditation without food and water. Eventually this demonstration itself spoke much louder than the appearance of his lack of experience or young age. Still there are those that to recognize the Power and Purity of Maha Sambodhi Dharma Sangha Guru's (as He is now called) message, teachings, and pathway.

You may be in your 40's but folks may not be able to recognize the truth you speak to them   Even with such an extreme demonstration as the Avatar Maha Sambodhi Dharma Sangha Guru made at age 16, some are still unable to recognize and they try to explain it away as a hoax or scam.

So really all that you can do is unhook your own mind from being attached to whether others can understand or hear what you Know, so that you may always have peace anyways. Because there will just always be some who will not be able to see through the conditioning of their own minds whether it be in regard to age or any other APPEARANCE of DIFFERENCE... Focus on your pathway and Be the Living Example of the Truth you wish to share or inspire others to follow.

If you feel a burning desire to relieve suffering in the world, then:

How can you best be of service and help; by drowning yourself in samsara (ocean of suffering)?   Or, by Realizing the Ultimate Freedom (Moksha) and building a bridge from samsara with the example of your life to the Safety of the Shore of Freedom (Illumined Awareness and Wisdom)?

Realizing the Essence of, and Connecting to the Guru. Purifying the Mind, and Realizing the Truth in the Heart

As before mentioned, it has been said in the ancient writings of the sages that the True Meaning of the Guru is difficult to reach even in Meditation.   This is very subtle realization and understanding like what has been called Secret in the Yogic teachings.   What is called the most secret knowledge is not necessarily because it should not be told.   Instead it is subtle Knowledge that cannot be conveyed only by words.   This subtle "silent" Knowing must be directly encountered within.

As a direct method of directly discovering this super subtle Knowledge of the Guru, the author has been guided to share the instructions which were passed to a friend and fellow sangha member by his Guru, Maha Sambodhi Dharma Sangha Guru.

This friend of the author has completely surrendered himself to Maha Sambodhi Dharma Sangha Guru as his Sadguru. The complete transformation in him since the 9 years ago when we first met is a living testament to the Great Power of Maha Sambodhi Dharma Sangha Guruji.

Early on in meeting Guruji, he was given these instructions. Maha Sambodhi Dharma Sangha Guru told him: "Contemplate Who is the Guru and What can the Guru do to purify the mind. When the mind is purified then look into the heart with purity and find the Truth. When It is found, one knows that the Truth is not meant for only oneself but is showered upon every living being in Creation."

This contemplation of "Who is the Guru, and What can the Guru do." will purify the mind and help one to directly realize the Guru Essence or Principle (Tattva). This contemplation can be started by simply repeating in the mind like a mantra "Who is the Guru and What can the Guru do?". But one should also move into contemplating beyond just thinking in words. To look with one's *Seeing* Power in the way of inquiry to consider really who is the Guru, and what can the Guru do.

This Purity of the mind which will be attained, is not to be thought of as something moral, or religious, like there are impure thoughts, and pure thoughts. Instead, the purity of the mind advised by the Masters for Realization is a complete and total clarity of mind. To be able to suspend or detach from All mental noise of ideas, thoughts, concepts etc. Otherwise we will only *see* the "clouds" of these many attachments within the mind, or have muddled seeing through the filter or this mental noise. That is why that Sages have advised that we cannot realize the Truth without first purity of mind, we will see only the relative truths or mistaken beliefs of our own mind.

After attaining a purity of mind, Maha Sambodhi Dharma Sangha Guru had advised to then go into the Heart. Within the Heart to look to *see* and directly encounter the Truth. These are very simple, but very complete and powerful instructions. If one genuinely follows these instructions it will certainly be life changing, and can be considered a complete method for purifying the mind through the Direct Connection with the Guru within.

When one directly connects with the Essence of the Guru within the Heart, they can receive guidance directly from That Omnipresent and Omniscient Super Intelligence. As the friend who relayed these instructions from Maha

Sambodhi Dharma Sangha Guruji also says. Now that he has nurtured a direct Connection to the Guru in his Heart over the 9 years since being given these instructions, he says any time he encounters a challenge or uncertain difficulty, he can connect directly to the Guru in his Heart and receive guidance or a solution.

Surrender

Give "yourself" up completely to the Pathway (Marga) of Harmony/Wholeness of Being (Dharma), to the Illumined One Being and Principle (Tattva) of Awakening (Gu Ru - the Light which Reveals and dispels the darkness of Ignorance), and Unity of Life as One (Love/Realization). Whoever we may think ourselves to be, it is all thinking, and all thought is *seen*. The thought that we are the doer, enjoyer, or sufferer of actions, body, or mind is also *seen*. Who believes this thought? Thus, surrender whatever you are doing, surrender it to the Whole...

Receiving the Upadesha (Advice) of Awakening, make efforts in the direction of Sadhana whenever you know the way to go. But don't identify as the doer of this. "Give yourself" up to the Super Intelligent Illumination of the Whole Supreme Being.   Call it forth in your sadhana directly like a channel.   That all your actions or appearance of efforts will be directed by the Super Intelligent Harmony (Dharma) of the Whole.   In Love (All Life as One), the *Seer Sees* Only this Super Intelligent Divine Being at all times and everywhere.

This body belongs in Harmony of the Whole.   Logically, intelligently it belongs in Service of the Whole.   Acting in division of the Whole is ignorance...   How can this body be said to belong to this thought "mine"?

Acting in Love (*Seeing* All Life as One) to Serve Harmony of Being, is Intelligence, and Knowing.   It is the Ability to *See* a bigger picture and *See* how it all fits together, and what it means!   Instantly, without even having to think about it, by direct connection of the Super Intelligence of Being.   One Being (All Beings) ... Do you See, how this all fits together?

Yoga is an Omniscient Unity of Being.   The mind sees two, Moon, Sun in Yogam they are One.   You want to attain Yoga?   Surrender all appearances to the Super Intelligent Light of Illumined Being.

Whatever "you" are doing, surrender it.   Don't take some pride in thinking you are the doer.   Or, some "spiritual" person.   Don't be fooled by thoughts of being better than someone or "superior" because of some "Awakening". Surrender in Love (All Life as One - the Divine Being). This is Real Devotion! Saying even just a few kind words to someone can be more powerful than "sadhana" puffed up with pride.

When you pray, pray for the Super Intelligence to completely act through "your" body for the Service of the Harmony of the Whole (Dharma). When doing mantra *see* the mantra manifesting the Super Intelligence of the Omniscient Being merging through all the faculties of Being for the Service of the Harmony of the Whole Omnipresent Being (Awakened Awareness). Surrender to allow that Principle (Tattva) of Awakening and Walking the Way (Marga) of Harmony (Dharma, Enlightenment, and Love {One}) to work through this Life for That Whole.

When we all align in Super Intelligent Harmony like this our Karma (Actions and Work) will powerfully co-create a True Heavenly Realm here even on Earth. This is the Intelligence, and Realization of Love.

Take for example what you may know from Love of your Family. A child, or Best Friend, Parents, whoever brings a feeling of Love. There is a natural inclination to the sacrifice of selfishness, and the intelligence of making an effort with the resources in Life to serve the well-being (Harmony) of the loved one.

Imagine what we could create with the Harmony of the Whole in Love, all acting in the Intelligence of Service to That One. Loving and Revering One Divine Being at all times, in all places and everywhere in all beings! Let us all surrender to the Super Intelligent Awakening of That One. Whatever we are doing.

Let us surrender to the Pathway (Marga) of Harmony/Wholeness of Being (Dharma), to the Illumined One Being and Principle (Tattva) of Awakening (Gu Ru - the Light which Reveals and dispels the darkness of Ignorance), and Unity of Life as One (Love/Realization).

That is what is happening, when we do outer sadhana of prostrations. Bowing and lowering the head before the image (murti) of Divinity. Whether an appearance of a living guru, or a stone, or a picture, a mountain, a river, a mouse. We are giving up what we are not, for the Truth of the Wholeness of Being. For those who may have wondered. And, those who may have not understood the principle of the Guru which syllables mean in Sanskrit (an Ancient phonetic language) the Light of the Awakened Intelligence which thus dispels the appearance of all ignorance.

Harmony of the Whole (Dharma)

Dharma gets misunderstood in many ways. It is often thought of as duty, or religion, or a set of rules. It's not that it isn't these things either, but it's not. Dharma is the support of the Universe and Infinity. Dharma is the Harmony with and of Wholeness of Being. The Harmony which is Dharma, is maintained by the Super Intelligence of the Whole. It is not philosophy... Dharma is in all actions and beyond all actions or doership.

If Dharma is a set of "rules" it is the policy of Intelligence which thus acts in Harmony with the Whole. If it is a "religion" it is the worship of Love (All Life as One), the Wholeness of Being (All Beings as One). If Dharma is your "duty", it is the natural role you play (when in Intelligence) in Harmony with your spouse, your parents or children, your community, your world, the Universe/infinity, the Whole of Life.

Dharma is Love (All Life as One)!

You are never Alone! We are All-One... We are Inevitably all interlinked as One Human Family, and with All Beings through Consciousness & Energy.

Do not accept philosophies promoting division, anger,

disagreement, or fighting among ourselves etc...

Realize and Understand that those media programs, stories, concepts, belief systems, leaders etc. which are promoting or spreading ideas which divide do not work for your best interest.

WE are VERY POWERFUL! When we realize our Unity and WORK TOGETHER in HARMONY (Dharma) we can rapidly bring about a TRUE AGE of PEACE and PROSPERITY.

Dividing our Hearts and Minds both internally and externally is a strategy of war. Divided not only are we weak, easy to conquer and control, but in ignorance we become our own enemies defeating our own World Family/Sangha and the right of all for Peace, Well Being, and Prosperity.

RETURN to the UNITY of LOVE! Don't believe you have reason to be angry or hateful towards anyone, if so, you are being deceived. Doesn't matter if they are a different sex, color, belief system, rich, poor, from another "country" etc. They are the same inherent LIGHT of LIFE FORCE, CONSCIOUSNESS & ENERGY as you. You are literally doing onto yourself as you do to others. Be a friend and kind to yourself, CHOOSE to act within the POWER of LOVE!

ALL of THE LOVE of the GREAT INFINITE WE is WITH

YOU ALWAYS!

The most powerful Sadhana you can ever do is Love. Apply it to your "Sangha" - community. As in allow yourself to apply a Pure Vision in Love where you see only the highest Divine Potential alive in everyone. See everyone as your chosen Divinity. Rather than dividing the seen (your vision) projecting judgement or "un-enlightened" beings, hold everyone in such a powerful uplifting Love that even once "ignorant" beings realize that Stainless Immortal Truth of Being called Self-Knowledge and also called Love...

When a Saint like Neem Karoli Baba was asked why or how he could possibly love and serve EVERYONE so unconditionally, N.K.B. replied that he saw only God everywhere.

This is very simple but Powerful Truth of Love (All Life as One) and Service! In this way the world could be transformed rapidly into a True Thriving Age of Peace and Prosperity by the powerful Work of One Humanity in Harmony (Dharma)...

Energy Transmissions, Attunements, Prayers, & Decrees

Om. All Obstacles Now Removed.
Opening the Gateways,
Calling in the Presence & Super Intelligent Light
Radiance of All Perfected Masters Combined.
For Full Awakening & Liberation
Concentrate the Way (Satya Parameshti Dharma Marga)
in the Potency of a Shaktipat Seed!
Received by whoever now reads...

[Take a deep breath in and release, open to receive]

Om Sarva Siddhar Jyoti Om
Om Sarva Param Atma Guru Jyoti Om
Om Parameshti Guru Jyoti Om
Om Satya Parameshti Dharma Marga Pradaayinyai Namah.

* * *

Illumined Intention of all Perfected Masters Combined,
Seeds of Enlightenment Dispersed on Winds of Compassion,
Burning Brilliant Blazing Flame of Realization Light The Way,
In Awareness, Presence, Stillness, Clarity of *Seeing* Now Shine!

* * *

Blaze Alchemical Love Flame of Freedom!
Love- Burning Searing Flame of Transformation,
Clear away all blockages to this Blissful feeling of Love,
Love for Self in All as One!
Bottomless Mystery of Infinity
Bound together by the impeccable freedom of Love!

* * *

AUM
May All Beings Know Peace!
Healing!
Ultimate Freedom!
Maha Moksha, the essential Nature, Immortal
Essence of Self Knowledge (Love) overflowing
throughout all Humanity...
So Be It!
This prayer multiplied 1,008,000,000 times every
time it is seen. AUM

* * *

OM,
Om Ganapati Om.
All Obstacles Removed!
Opening the Gateways.
Under the Guidance
of my Healing & Guidance Team.
In Perfect Harmony with

My Highest Pathway of Wholeness & Harmony.
All the Infinite Possibilities & Resources
of the Super Intelligent Divine Energy!
The Perfected Master Self "Integration Point" In
which All of the Life Stream is Integrated as all aspects,
and Moments in One Perfect Wholeness of Being!
Calling Upon the "Celestial Healer" Like an
Archetype as the Source of All Healing Knowledge,
Modalities, and Energies!
Bringing forth whatever Is needed for Balance of
Holistic Health and Well-Being,
From the Infinite Possibilities of Pure Energy (Maha
Shakt)!
That whatever can Be Received, Released, Balanced,
Harmonized, in Safety, with Gentleness, and
Nurturing Loving Support,
At this Time, Sacred Moment of Now.
With Ongoing Integration under the Guidance of
Super Intelligent Energy
and, Radiant Light of Perfected Masters,
and Perfected Mastery of the Entire Life Stream as
One Seeing.
Life Force in Balance, Harmony, Wholeness, and
Super Intelligent Maintenance for True Health and
Well Being.

Divine Mother, and Supreme Lord
Hear our Prayers for the relieving of suffering,
Nurturing Wholeness, Health, Well-Being,
Illumination,
Total Freedom, Liberation, Light Body of Bliss.
Sealing the Field in High Frequency Super
Intelligent Light of this Being's greatest capacity of
Harmony, Wholeness, Health, and Wellness!
With a protective Blazing Brilliant Blue White Light
like an Armor, so that nothing of harmful, or negative
intention ever manifests within this Life!
Om Namah Shivaaya
Automatically Multiplied 1 Billion 8 Million Times!
OM

* * *

Aum Namah Shivaya Automatically Multiplied
1,008,000,000 Times in All who see this!
For the Purpose of lending an incredible boost of
Energy, Shakti.
To break any habitual tendencies
that are no longer useful.
Plugging energy leaks, dissolving all obstacles,

Overcoming all limits and boundaries...

Aum Namah Shivaya x 1,008,000,000
A BOOST of POWER
to assist You
to create the Life of Your Highest Peace, Fulfillment,
and Total Harmony!

Aum Namah Shivaya x 1,008,000,000
That this Ocean of Energy
may guide any and all
shifts, evolution, and transmutation to occur
with grace and ease...
So that this "work" may actually be pure
enjoyment.

Aum Namah Shivaya x 1,008,000,000
An incredible Boost of Energy Now!
Clarity, Impeccability, Truth, Simplicity, LOVE.
Miracles occur Daily!

Aum Namaha Sivaaya x Infinity
No limit to the power and support to Live Ultimate
Freedom!

Maitri Mangalam Astu
Shantir Astu
Maha Moksha Astu!

* * *

Open channel, dazzling bright,
Super Intelligent Cosmic Light!
Inspiration, Realization, Liberation,
Ultimate Freedom!

* * *

7 Param Atma Guru's revealed by Maha Sambodhi Dharma Sangha Guru, Immediately Blaze Your Brilliant Powerful Presence Around and Throughout this body/mind/heart Energy Field!

Cleanse and Release any and all Harmful Cords, Energetic Parasites, Implants, Negative or Trouble Making Entities.

Provide constant and continuous Protection & Guidance to remain in Harmony, Illumined Awareness, Super Intelligence, and Firmly on the Satya Dharma Marga.

Thank you, Thank you, Thank you for your unfailing Power, Support, and Presence in this Life!

Love (All Life as One)!

* * *

May all obstacles to pure Love dissolve
naturally, easily, effortlessly,
that all may swim in the fulfillment of Unconditional
Love for All!

* * *

The Light of Awareness is Love.

The Energy/Force of Life is Love.

The Knowledge of the Self is Love.

The Goal and Source of Life is Love...

* * *

Divine All Pervasive Parameshti Guru Tattva!
Deep Within,
We the Appearance of All Beings, Now Call to Thee!
Show Grace! Divine Protection!
Remove, Overcome, Blaze, Burn, Cut Through,
Purify All Obstacles and Forces in Opposition to
Illumined Awareness!
Bestow Clarity to Follow the Way of Harmony
[Dharma]!

* * *

Parameshti Siddheshvari Svarupini, all form, everywhere and everything, all intensities and appearances of realities, all possibilities and experiences of Being. Kshamasya Karo, Dayaa Karo, Krpa Karo, charanam Karo - forgive "me" for all ignorance of divisions, conflicts and errors.

Knowing that this appearance of "me" is also only thee Infinite Divine Maha Maya Shakti, and that "I" am only blundering as a fool attempting to serve thee. Always reveal your Divine Essence and Nature in Crystal Clarity, Potency, and Presence of the Moment.

Parameshti Marga Pradinyai Namaha, Parameshti Siddha Gyan Pradinyai Namaha, Parameshti Siddha Marga Darshana Pradinyai Namaha - Lead us Directly on the Supreme Pathway, Grant the Supreme Knowledge of Perfection, Reveal Directly Before us the Ultimate Pathway of the Perfect Expression of Awareness.

Thank You, Thank You, Thank You,

Divine Mother Infinity - All Energy!

* * *

Ancestor Prayer at the Time of Memorial or Funeral

Om.
Primordial Pure Stainless Awareness,
Supreme Lord and the Source of Consciousness and Love!

Thank you Mother Father God for your Gentle but Powerful Guiding Grace Light, Now with our Beloved Ancestor, we knew as _____ [Name of departed]_____.

This name, body, and life story is cast aside like an outworn blanket now... It's stories and desires are completely fulfilled. Remembered as a Great and Inspiring [Man/Woman] in so many ways, there is nothing to regret as you move forward to your Highest Goal's fulfillment, Heavenly Existence and Wholeness (Holyness).

We continue to receive your Guiding Light here, as living presence in our hearts, within the human world. And, likewise we promise to fulfill our Duty to repay your Loving Service by realizing our own highest potential, and Life.

We will remember to embrace the fullness of Life. And, continue to pray that we may be able to live in balance, strong, peaceful, content and fulfilled in the essence of Life. All of our lineage, ancestors, ourselves, our descendants, be now aligned, harmonized, purified, and guided in Divine Grace, Wisdom, and Love!

In Gratitude we celebrate your life. In great Expansive Wisdom and penetrating intuitive insight into Life, we celebrate this new joyful chapter in your eternal life. May Supreme Divinity and Victorious Enlightened Master's guide you in fulfilling your Life Stream's True Desires. Abiding in heavenly realms, enjoying celestial bliss, or skillful and strategic rebirth in a joyful and fulfilling lifetime on Earth... May your Soul's Greatest Fulfillment be Divinely Guided and Swiftly Realized.

In Love and Gratitude beyond words... Divine One, Thanks for Everything, Thanks for Being! We owe you our lives! We will do our Duty and discover just what is the essence of this Life, and Live it!

Love!

Om, Hreem...

Conclusion

The pathway of sadhana can be simplicity itself. It is simply the giving up of the untrue for the ever present and immortal Truth. The mind has infinite possibilities of angles and views. One of the main obstacles is that we have often formed a habit of seeing the world only through the mind. Thus, many issues that we may have in Life, or apparent obstacles on the Way of Harmony and Wholeness, are simply imagined within the mind. Step back as a pure witness of the mind itself. Look for the source of thought and all perception. Don't unnecessarily believe all that you think...

The Awakened and Ever Pure Awareness is ever-present and omnipotent. The Truth of Being is already the Reality whether known or unknown. Be Alert! Be Aware! The Supreme is ever present! The nature of the Pathway and Enlightenment is not a philosophy. Words are not enough! Follow the pointers here now and contemplate directly into the Nature of Being, and all perception.

If this is understood it can only be applied. It must be "Lived". Put into a new way of action. But even to describe this as "action" is not sufficient. All the world is engaged in action. This is the "not-doing" of action. The body and or mind are not idle. They are aligned in the impeccability of (Dharma) Harmony with and Service to the Whole. The only thing that is missing is "you"! Or who you may have been dreaming, imagining, or thinking was you... The Self, One and the Same in All, does not fade.

You may feel free to write Darshan with any questions, anytime. As long as there is the time and availability, Darshan will be happy to serve in any way that he can! May you see and feel the Support of Love (All Life as One). By the Super Intelligent Guidance of All Life as One (Love) may your life flow in Harmony with the Whole (Dharma).

Namaste & Pranams Divine Universal World Sangha!

With Love, Darshan Baba

More Moksha Gyan Books by Darshan Baba for you to Read:

- **Free "A Self Attunement: Maha Moksha Healing" PDF eBook version** available to download or print. Shaktipat & Healing Energy Transmission through 10-minute affirmational reading! Can be a Daily Practice. Paperback sells at $15.95 list price, but you can get this eBook version free now, to start reading today!

If you don't have it *already,* go get it now --->>https://siddha-international.weebly.com/fresubtleenergybook.html

- Cosmic Consciousness & Healing with the Quantum Field: A Guide to Holding Space Facilitating Healing, Attunements, Blessings, and Empowerments for Self and Others

- True Sadhana: Siddha Yoga (Perfection of Yoga) Manifesting Within the Seeker

- Yoga Sadhana of the Mother of the Universe: A

Guide to Wholeness Through the Divine Feminine

- Babaji's Manasa Yoga of Moksha

See all the Moksha Gyan Books by Darshan Baba on Amazon now:
https://amazon.com/author/moksha

Moksha Gyan Music

Available on Amazon as Compact Disc:
- Infinite Light
- Yoga Sadhana of the Mother of the Universe CD Companion

Some titles available on your favorite music streaming & download sites like iTunes..

All Moksha Gyan Music titles can be checked out & streamed online for free at:
https://moksha-gyan-music.bandcamp.com

Siddha Life Mastery Online Courses

- Intro & Experience of Subtle Energy

- Ultimate Subtle Energy Mastery Course

- Ultimate Meditation Course: Siddha Jyoti & Nada Dhyana Kriya Initiation and Practice Instruction

Sign up FREE for Your Siddha Life Mastery online course now go to: https://siddha-life-mastery.com

Siddha Subtle Energy Medicine & Shaktipat with Darshan Baba

Sign up for your distance Siddha Subtle Energy Transmission here:

https://siddha-international.weebly.com/siddha-subtle-energy-healing-shaktipat.html

To arrange for in person session, intensive training, healing retreat, group session/training/retreat, etc. Email: omnamahshivaya8@gmail.com

Want Darshan Baba as a Guest Speaker, Trainer, or Presenter at your Event?

Contact Darshan Baba by email:
omnamahshivaya8@gmail.com
Or by Phone: +15756138137